Making Sense of Trauma

Dr Nigel C. Hunt is an academic psychologist – Associate Professor in the School of Community Health Sciences, University of Nottingham. He is also Reader in Traumatic Stress Studies at the University of Helsinki, Finland. He obtained his PhD, entitled 'The long-term psychological effects of war experience', at the University of Plymouth. Since then he has written several books, including *Memory, War and Trauma* (Cambridge) and numerous articles in academic journals and elsewhere, mostly on the subject of traumatic stress. He conducts research with war veterans and other traumatized people in a variety of contexts and in many different countries.

Sue McHale is Senior Lecturer in Biological Psychology at Sheffield Hallam University. She obtained her PhD at the University of Plymouth, and has interests in stress, coping and emotion, and in the effects of drugs on behaviour. She has written many articles in academic journals and elsewhere.

Dr Hunt and Dr McHale have jointly written two books for Sheldon Press: *Coping with Alopecia* (2004) and the companion volume to this book, *Understanding Traumatic Stress* (2010). They have have also written several academic articles, mainly on memory and on the psychosocial impact of alopecia.

D0495842

Overcoming Common Problems Series

Selected titles

A full list of titles is available from Sheldon Press,
36 Causton Street, London SW1P 4ST and on our website at
www.sheldonpress.co.uk

Overcoming Common Problems Series

Overcoming Common Problems Series

Overcoming Common Problems

Making Sense of Trauma

How to tell your story

DR NIGEL C. HUNT
DR SUE McHALE

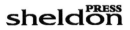

First published in Great Britain in 2012

Sheldon Press
36 Causton Street
London SW1P 4ST
www.sheldonpress.co.uk

Copyright © Nigel C. Hunt and Sue McHale 2012

All rights reserved. No part of this book may be reproduced or
transmitted in any form or by any means, electronic or mechanical,
including photocopying, recording, or by any information storage and
retrieval system, without permission in writing from the publisher.

The author and publisher have made every effort to ensure that the
external website and email addresses included in this book are correct and
up to date at the time of going to press. The author and publisher are not
responsible for the content, quality or continuing accessibility of the sites.

British Library Cataloguing-in-Publication Data
A catalogue record for this book is available from the British Library

ISBN 978-1-84709-147-5

Typeset by Fakenham Prepress Solutions, Fakenham, Norfolk NR21 8NN
Printed in Great Britain by Ashford Colour Press
Subsequently digitally printed in Great Britain

Produced on paper from sustainable forests

Contents

1

Introduction

We all know that there are events in life that are so distressing that life itself becomes very difficult. Some of us experience war, whether as a soldier or as a civilian. Some live through natural disasters such as earthquakes or volcanic eruptions. Some live through manmade disasters such as the sinking of a ship or a terrorist outrage, or at a more personal level a devastating car crash, rape and sexual abuse, or a serious illness. Most of us at some point lose important members of our family or our friends, or have to try and help someone through the experience of an illness such as cancer. Some people cope very well with these experiences; others do not cope so well. We are all very different. Some people rely heavily on their family and friends to help them; others try to get through the problems by themselves. What all these events (and others) have in common is that they can be considered 'traumatic'.

A traumatic event is fundamentally disruptive to a person's life. It shatters one's personal belief system, has a terrible effect on the ability to control one's emotions, and can significantly change one's behaviour and interactions with other people. We all react differently to these events, and there is certainly no more or less appropriate response. At the worst extreme there are people who develop what is known as post-traumatic stress disorder (PTSD), which will be discussed in Chapter 2. Perhaps the majority of people will have some bad dreams or sad or fearful thoughts, but will be able to put the event to one side and get on with life. Others – perhaps the luckier ones – may spontaneously learn from the event and will change the way they think about the world, perhaps in a positive manner. These three basic response styles are all common, but what narrative does is try and help people to come to terms with their experiences in a positive manner – or at least avoid the worst problems such as PTSD.

What is narrative?

Narrative is what we all do to varying extents in most situations in which we find ourselves. We are all storytellers. We make sense of the world we live in, we create meaning, and we explain things that have happened to us and others. We largely do this in an informal manner, chatting with friends, writing a diary, sending text messages, interpreting the news. Some of us spend more time doing formal narratives. A teacher will use a lesson to put across a narrative, whether that is about the plays of Shakespeare or the best way to construct a bridge from empty toilet rolls. A book is a formal narrative, consisting of a number of chapters that in the end tell a story.

Types of personal narrative, from the trivial to the autobiography

Our narratives work at different levels, from those that concern something that happened at work or school through to the higher-level life narratives that we use to explain our lives generally. At one level, we get new narratives every day. When we get home from work or study we might tell family members about what happened. This won't be in the detail of 'At 9 a.m. I did such and such and at 9.30 a.m. I did so and so,' etc., but we focus on the more important and interesting parts of the day. We might tell a story about someone at work who had a problem and how that problem was solved. There might have been an interesting visitor. We might have heard some juicy gossip, the type of thing that is meant to be private but everyone knows it: 'Don't tell anyone but Joe has been having an affair with Josephine for the last four months. His wife still doesn't know anything about it.' This is hopefully not an everyday story, but you get the gist. These stories add to one's repertoire of stories, which themselves build together to make a larger whole. This in the end is our autobiography, the stories of our lives and of those we interact with. We create and recreate our autobiography continually. Memory consists not of a large number of accurate recollections about what has happened to us over the years, but our current interpretation of these events. It is about our personal *interpretations* of ourselves and others.

This idea that our life narratives change and develop is crucial to understanding the role of narrative in our lives. It is a key part of our identity, what it means to be 'me'. It is also important for our mental health. For example, most of us are – most of the time – reasonably happy or contented with our lives. A few of us are discontented and may experience symptoms of depression. At the other end of the scale are the fortunate few who are very happy and have an extremely optimistic view of the world. The group to which we belong depends on many things, including personality, coping styles, friends and family, and what happens to us in the world. One of the key differences, however, is that depressed people interpret their lives differently from the people who are not depressed. Let's say two people have similar lives: good things happen, bad things happen, relationships vary from poor to excellent, and work is acceptable but not fantastic. The person who is not depressed tends to focus on the more positive aspects of life, the events that make her happy, the behaviour of people who help her deal with problems, or having a good social life. The depressed person focuses on different events: on not having enough money in the bank, the wayward relative, or the fact that he is overweight. The differences between these two people are the way they construct their narratives about themselves, about other people and about the world. The first person focuses on the positive and develops a positive narrative; the second focuses on the negative and develops a depressive narrative.

In the end, we are constantly developing and adapting our autobiographies to account for what is happening in our lives and relationships. The depressed person can develop a more positive narrative by learning to focus on more positive events. Unfortunately there is another complication. We do not have a single life story; we adapt and change it not just for ourselves but also for others, for those who are listening to us.

Audience

Narratives nearly always have an audience. Whatever story we are trying to tell, however we are projecting ourselves to others and to the world, the narrative is built on the assumption of an audience.

It does not matter whether the narrative is in a written form – a book, a letter, an email, a comment on a social networking site – or is in a verbal form – talking with friends and relatives – or is just the result of sitting and thinking about a topic: in each one, the assumption of the audience is paramount. It is simple to show the importance of the audience. Think about the story of your life: about what has happened to you and the way it has affected your development. Think about the good things; think about the things you may be embarrassed about. Then put yourself in the position of telling your life story to different people. Assume you are a married male – happily married – with a good job that involves working closely with colleagues and subordinates, and also that you have some good friends (or use your own scenario). If people from these different categories asked you about your life you would be likely to tell them different stories. You may not want your wife to know about certain previous girlfriends. You may not want your work colleagues to know about the time you got a police record for hooliganism as an adolescent. You may be more honest with one close friend than another friend. The point is, you want to portray yourself in a particular way. This links to what we said about depression earlier. There is no single way to describe your past. It is interpreted both by how you see yourself now and by how you want others to see you. Inevitably, we have many life stories, all incomplete, all biased in one way or another depending on how we want to see ourselves and how we want others to see us.

The importance of the audience is seen when someone is traumatized. Not only is that person traumatized, but the effects are seen among the people who surround him or her: friends and relations, they too are often badly affected. Sometimes they hear tales of horror; on other occasions it may be fear or anger resulting from what happened to the traumatized person; it may be the anger of the traumatized person; or it may be that they simply do not know how to respond to what has happened, how to help, whether to talk about it or not.

Traumatic events

The problem with traumatic events is that they fundamentally disrupt our life narratives. They destroy the meaning of our lives, what we think of ourselves, of other people, of the world around us. As mentioned, trauma affects not only the person's life, it affects those around, family and friends, work colleagues and neighbours. The effects of a traumatic experience can be very wide-ranging. People who are severely affected may require not only psychological help but drug therapy from a GP or psychiatrist.

The traumatic memory is key to understanding psychological trauma. A traumatic memory of an event can consist of cognitive, affective (emotional) and behavioural elements. When a traumatic memory is triggered by a reminder of the event, the traumatized person may automatically respond with negative emotions (such as fear, anger or horror), negative behaviours (such as aggression) and negative cognitions (such as negative beliefs about other people). One of the interesting features about traumatic memories is that they have the effect of making the person 'stuck' in the past; traumatized people are unable to think away from the time of the traumatic event, and so cannot get on with their lives. If a person is stuck in the past, it is going to be difficult to live life fully in the present and through his or her relationships. The resolution of trauma involves being able to deal with the traumatic memory and enabled to live life to the full again. The development of post-trauma narratives is important in this process. Indeed, it is critical to this process, because all forms of therapy involve the development of narratives – even drug therapy, which when used appropriately can help people think more clearly about what has happened to them, or can enable them to benefit from psychotherapy. Prescribed drugs do not work when they are used inappropriately and stop the person from thinking clearly. While there may be a temporary benefit to this state of mind, in that it may give the person respite from the horror, in the end he or she needs to find some way of engaging with the world again.

People affected by traumatic experiences generally want to make sense of those experiences. This can occur in a number of ways: through the passage of time, through therapy or counselling, through talking to friends and family, or simply by thinking about it or writing about it. All of these involve – or are – narrative. Narrative is about stories, the development and relating of stories, a means of telling oneself or others about an experience. It involves making meaning from the event, putting it in context, explaining why it happened and the effect it had on oneself. Once this meaning-making is complete (if it can ever be complete), a person is more able to live with the memory of the event, and any symptoms may diminish.

Why this book?

The purpose of this book is to describe the processes involved in narrative or storytelling, with a range of techniques that can be used to generate stories or meaning. We are all different and use many ways to create and develop stories. What is a good technique for one person will not work for another, so the book introduces many different approaches. In the end, to be human is to be able to narrate and to narrate is to be human, so using narrative to deal with traumatic memories is a natural approach to sorting out one's problems. We construct narratives continually, about all aspects of our lives. As already stated, narratives are fundamentally social. They exist to inform ourselves and others about something. For that reason if we are to talk about narrative we must also discuss the audience, the people who provide social support for those affected by traumatic events.

This idea of social support is important. We have a tendency to dismiss it, but as human beings we are dependent upon social support. This is the name psychologists use when talking about the role friends, family and colleagues play in helping us when there is something wrong. We rely on others, and we should rely on others. Other people help us develop and change our narratives and make sense of the world; they comfort us through problems and are necessary for the development of meaning. People who are affected by trauma can benefit by having others to help them rebuild the meaning in their lives, particularly because trauma can be such a deep cut, a cut that can hinder the ability of people to help construct narratives. One purpose of the book is to provide techniques to help with this process.

In the end, the book is about narrative healing. It is about the development of stories that help people deal with their problems, make sense of situations and – where possible – grow psychologically and spiritually from what has happened to them.

The various chapters of the book present different methods of narrative development. Some people like to write, others to talk, others to draw or paint. These are covered in the respective chapters. There are also case studies which show how people use techniques to help themselves. These show not only how narrative techniques work, but also how they can go wrong. They are designed to help you further understand the importance of narratives and how you can apply techniques to help yourself.

Chapter 2 explores the nature of traumatic and stressful events in more detail. It is all very well to talk about traumatic events, but what are they? What is the fundamental nature of a traumatic event? What do we mean by PTSD and the range of other responses that people have to such events? In the medical world, these responses are seen as mental disorders, though they are intelligible as appropriate responses to terrible situations.

Chapter 3 explores the common ways in which we deal with distressing events, through coping and social support. What are the personal and interpersonal processes that are going on when we try to deal with such events? There has been a lot of research about the notion of coping, and we know that people have different coping styles, some of which are more effective than others. It is normal to ponder on something that is bothering us, and it is just as normal to avoid situations that remind us of something that bothers us. To some extent we can control the ways we cope, but coping is also a basic personality characteristic that should be taken into account when thinking about narratives.

Chapter 4 focuses on the more positive outcomes of traumatic experience and the utility of positive narratives. While it may seem to you that there are no positive aspects, there is now a great deal of evidence that many people experience what we call post-traumatic growth: that is, the life-threatening nature of the traumatic experience has made them think differently about the world. Perhaps they focus more on living a 'good life', or maybe the nearness of death has made them better able to appreciate life. It may make them get more out of their relationships with friends and family. In some way, even though the traumatic event is tragic, the person's life narrative has been enhanced and improved as an outcome of that event.

Chapter 5 continues the discussion about narrative, focusing more on the normality of storytelling, the way we use stories all the time and the basic rules about what makes a good story. It brings in the idea that the main story we have is our own auto-biography. It is this autobiography that is undermined by the experience of trauma.

Chapter 6 provides a warning: working through the exercises in this book, dealing with your traumatic experiences through narrative development, can be upsetting. It is important that you have the necessary personal resources, including support from friends and family, before you embark on the process.

We then move on to the chapters that are specifically concerned with providing means of help, known as Guided Narrative Techniques (GNTs), which are the means of guiding you in making meaning out of your experiences. These GNTs are designed to help you with structuring your narratives. There are a number of different methods, not all involving writing, as you will see in the next chapters.

Chapter 7 is concerned with one of the most basic things we can do to help ourselves: going for a walk. The chapter emphasizes the value of walking, the way it enables us to think more clearly – or sometimes to avoid thinking. The chapter examines ways of thinking through our problems while walking alone, and of talking through them when walking with another person.

Chapter 8 is concerned with writing techniques. Writing has been proved to be immensely helpful for a lot of people. The simple act of writing about one's troubles is helpful. At one level it doesn't matter what is written, as the act of writing is the creation of a narrative. This chapter focuses on the range of techniques introduced by James Pennebaker, though many different researchers have used these ideas in different ways. Another method is derived from Narrative Exposure Therapy (NET), designed by Frank Neuner and colleagues a few years ago to help refugees deal with their traumatic memories. It is derived from both cognitive behavioural therapy

(CBT) and testimony therapy, and helps people tell their stories in a way that not only makes sense to them but could also be used as witness testimony against someone later indicted for war crimes. This is important because when we create narratives we often want a meaningful audience, not an artificial story. With NET, an individual is guided to tell his or her own story of the trauma, which is then written out, read back to the person and rewritten until the story is complete. We use a simplified personally administered version of the technique.

Chapter 9, 'Writing for and with others', is a short chapter that describes the benefits of writing with others, whether that is through traditional letters, emails or various forms of internet activity such as discussion forums and social networking sites. All are helpful to the traumatized person; all are useful means of providing support. The internet is particularly helpful, as forums and networking sites are often areas where people with similar experiences can share their understanding and exchange information.

Chapter 10, another short chapter, looks at how other people's more formal trauma narratives can be very useful. Books, poems, and plays are all extremely helpful for increasing our understanding of trauma. A description of the trauma of war or sexual abuse by someone who has been through such experiences again enhances our personal understanding. Novelists who write about traumatic events can also enhance our understanding, even if they have not been through these events themselves.

Chapter 11 explores art and narrative. While many people talk or write about their experiences, others use alternative methods. Many people – including children – have been helped by using art and narrative, by telling the story of the trauma through photographs, paintings and drawings. The event is depicted in any way the person wishes. A landscape can help, as shown by the photographs of Don McCullen – who started taking landscape photographs after he had finished taking photographs of war – or by the paintings of Paul Nash, who painted landscapes once he had got away from the battlefields of the First World War.

In Chapter 12 we move away from the individual troubled by traumatic memories to groups and communities. Groups of people who have shared an experience often get together to talk through what has happened and the meanings that the event has for them. Talking about your thoughts and feelings with a group of people with similar experiences can be very helpful. At the level of the larger community, stories about a shared event can also be gathered, discussed and made meaningful. While we are not suggesting you need to be involved in groups, if an opportunity arises then you could benefit from them.

Chapter 13 is a discussion about the limits of deriving your own meaning from your experiences and developing your own narratives, and discusses how sometimes you need a therapist to help you overcome your problems. While many people can help themselves or make effective use of their support networks, others cannot. In this chapter we outline some of the key professional therapies that are available, and also show how they help people to develop narratives.

Chapter 14 draws together the material presented in the earlier chapters and provides an overview of what has been covered. Finally, at the end of the book, Appendix A provides a set of measures that you can use to look at your own levels of traumatic stress, depression and anxiety and substance abuse, and also to look at how you cope and your levels of post-traumatic growth; Appendix B provides a table of options to help you when deciding which activity to use. Finally, we suggest some addresses you may find useful and give ideas for further reading.

We have written the book with this structure for a purpose, that it should be read cover to cover, but of course you do not have to do this. We have set it out so that the chapters can stand alone, but we recommend you read it in its entirety so that you understand the critical importance of storytelling, of narrative, with regard to most aspects of our lives, including dealing with traumatic stress. After all, the book itself is meant to be a narrative.

2

The nature of traumatic events

It is difficult to define what we mean by a traumatic event, because what is traumatic to one person is not traumatic to another. This immediately identifies a key issue – while the medical and psychological literature focuses on the effect a traumatic event has on a person, there can be no definition of what a traumatic event is, nor what the impact is on someone! An historical perspective gives us some insight into the varying nature of traumatic events.

The earliest research relating to traumatic stress concerned war. For centuries, people have recorded the psychological effects of war. If we read Homer's *Iliad* – written about 2,800 years ago about events that took place over 3,000 years ago – we can see the psychological effects of war. Achilles, the hero, clearly shows symptoms of what we would now call post-traumatic stress disorder (PTSD). He is distraught, he cannot think straight, he makes bad decisions; and then when his friend Patroclus dies he runs amok, kills his enemy Hector and abuses his body. In this, Achilles displays strong symptoms of PTSD. Again in ancient times, Herodotus records the story of a young man at the battle of Marathon who is found after the battle without any apparent wound, but who has lost the use of his legs and his eyes. He is paralysed in a way seen among many First World War veterans who experienced strong physical symptoms to the stress of war, and his blindness is perhaps attributable to the fright of seeing the horrors of the battlefield.

The twentieth century saw big changes in the way we look at traumatic stress. At the beginning of the First World War the concept of 'shellshock' was introduced. Men who had broken down in battle were thought to have had minor, sometimes invisible wounds, where a piece of shell or shrapnel had entered the brain and caused damage which led to these psychological problems. By the end of that war there was some understanding that the horrors of war could cause such symptoms. By the Vietnam War in the

1960s and 1970s it was recognized that war itself could cause psychological problems.

PTSD was introduced as a disorder in 1980. Initially it was based on the symptoms of the US veterans returning from the Vietnam War, but it wasn't long before people who had experienced other traumatic events were shown to be traumatized in a very similar way. Within the next decade research had been carried out with rape victims and victims of prolonged sexual abuse, and people who had experienced natural and manmade disasters, car accidents and other kinds of events. Though the events were very different, many of the symptoms were similar.

PTSD describes the main symptoms that people can experience after a traumatic event. These include being emotional after an event, having intrusive memories (those that you have no control over), avoiding reminders of the event, emotional numbing (not being able to feel emotions in the normal way) and physiological symptoms such as the inability to sleep or a heightened startle reaction. These are common symptoms after a traumatic event. Other common reactions are feelings of anxiety or depression, or drinking more than usual. There is nothing intrinsically wrong with any of these symptoms; experiencing them doesn't make you 'ill'. They are normal responses to a terrible experience.

Let's look at this in more detail. Traumatic events are often thought of as not happening to most of us – which is not true. While most of us will – hopefully – not experience war or a natural disaster, most of us experience things that cause us a great deal of pain. The death of a relative or a friend is something that is difficult to bear. We all find it difficult to come to terms with such a death.

One of the problems with psychology is that it can easily label people as being ill when they are not. If someone dies, or if we are in a traffic accident, or if there is a fire, it is inevitable that it will upset us. Think of the things listed earlier regarding post-traumatic stress disorder: the horrible memories, the desire to avoid thinking about what has happened, the bad dreams, the feeling of anxiety; while these are symptoms of post-traumatic stress disorder, they are also normal responses to terrible events. It would be unusual if, after a very stressful event, we didn't have bad dreams or feel anxiety. That does not mean that we are ill, that we need some sort of psychological treatment. While some people do need help, it is important to remember that just because you have negative thoughts and emotions, you are not mentally ill.

After a traumatic event, it is only a minority of people who experience serious psychological consequences that require some form of therapy; most of us get upset and learn to cope. One of the purposes of this book is to show that there are some good ways of coming to terms with a traumatic experience. That is not to deny the seriousness of how we feel and think after a terrible incident, nor the real consequences of that event, but we do need to look at how we can come to terms with it and move our lives forward.

What do we mean by a traumatic event?

Clinicians still dispute what is meant by a traumatic event. When PTSD was introduced in 1980, a traumatic event was an event 'outside the realm of normal human experience', and so was assumed to be something that didn't happen to most of us. There was a quick realization that this was wrong. Even if we just talk of war, many millions of people experience this every year; it is commonplace in many countries. It is now accepted that there are many types of traumatic event. Apart from war, these include rape and sexual abuse, road traffic accidents, the sudden unexpected death of a loved one, natural disasters, manmade disasters, and other forms of violence against the person. For an event to be traumatic it has to be profoundly upsetting at the time and involve threatened death or serious injury to oneself or others, or the actual death of others. There is, of course, flexibility in exactly what events count as traumatic, and experts will inevitably disagree about what constitutes a trauma. The main thing is that if an event is traumatic to you, it is traumatic.

Then what do we mean by 'traumatic'? Clearly, there has to be a threat to life and well-being. This threat has to be accompanied by emotions such as fear, helplessness or horror. There are huge individual differences about who will become traumatized after an event, and we cannot and should not assume people will be traumatized. The traumatized person not only goes through the event but experiences a fundamental breakdown of the way he or she thinks about things. Most of us usually have a fairly positive view about ourselves, other people and the world. A traumatizing event destroys these thoughts. After a traumatic event our positive narratives about the world are ruined, and we start to look at everything with fearful eyes, or we see the world as unsafe and people as frightening; we might look on ourselves as worthless, perhaps because of how we behaved or didn't behave during the traumatic event.

Of course, variations arise not only from differences between people but also from the type of event. Events such as natural disasters, which are not caused by people and tend to be single happenings, usually have less of a profound and complex effect than events that involve a perpetrator such as a rapist or murderer, or events that are complex, repeated and long-lasting, such as child sex abuse or war. Complex events can affect people more seriously, and are more difficult to come to terms with, than simple events not caused by a person. People are also more affected if they had no sense of control during the traumatic event. The soldier who fires his rifle is not as affected as the soldier who sits in a trench being fired on. The person who manages to help others climb out from a sinking ship is less affected than the people being helped out.

Nevertheless, it is not possible to predict who is going to be traumatized by a particular experience, nor to say that particular experiences will always lead to psychological problems. Psychological problems can emerge from a whole range of events. Jean was raped by her drunken husband and his friend late one night; that experience, perpetrated by the person who should have been protecting her, caused an utter breakdown in Jean's ability to trust anyone. John was in the pub with his mates when a gang walked in; one of them forced an argument with John's friend Barry, drew a knife and stabbed him to death. This was so unexpected that John and his friends didn't have time to respond before the gang had gone, but John felt guilty that he had not been able to protect Barry. Stacey was at home asleep when the house caught fire; she managed to escape but her two children died. Peter survived a car crash that killed his child. The cases are endless. What we are trying to do in this book is to show how you can try and come to terms with your experiences through making sense of what has happened.

Examples

Throughout the book we are going to use a number of case studies to illustrate the points we are trying to make. Here, we can see that the type of traumatic event can affect the kind of problems people experience.

The earthquake victim

On 12 May 2008 there was a serious earthquake in Sichuan province, China, that measured 8.0 on the Richter scale; it killed over 69,000 people and left 4.8 million people homeless. At the time of writing, around three years later, many people are still homeless and many continue to suffer as a result of losing family and friends or being injured. May Han is a typical example. May had lived all her life in a single village, was married and had one child. When the earthquake happened her husband was at work and her child at school; she was at home. The earthquake destroyed her home, but she escaped before it collapsed. Everything was chaos around her and her first thought was for her child. She ran along the road through the collapsed buildings only to find that the school was a heap of rubble. A number of children and adults were milling around, mostly looking confused. May frantically searched for her child, calling her name, asking the other children if they had seen her. No one had. She saw no one from her child's class. She went to where she thought the classroom was, but there was nothing left except rubble. Nevertheless she ran up to it and started clawing away at the concrete and the bricks, trying to get through, shouting her child's name. Others were there too, trying to help, trying to find their own children. No one else, it seemed, came to help. People stood around not knowing what to do; others knelt on the ground, or just lay there. May dug for what seemed like hours, achieving little, seeing no evidence of any buried child. Eventually rescue workers came along and gently led her away, sobbing, saying that they were going to dig now. They took her to a shelter where she stayed with a number of other mothers, none knowing how to comfort each other in their grief. May then thought about her husband, who would surely have come to look for her. What had happened to him? She asked people nearby if they knew what had happened to her husband's factory. No one knew anything. She went up to a nurse, who said she would try and find out – but the nurse was trying to find information for so many people. In the end May decided to look for herself. She again went through the ruined streets, this time to the nearby factory where her husband worked. It was cordoned off; she could see that this building too was destroyed. She asked a man who seemed to be in charge what had happened to the workers, and he told her that some had died and many had been injured and taken to hospital. She found out which hospital and again hurried through the streets. At the hospital she found people lying all over the ground outside – there was no room for them inside the building. At the reception desk she was turned away and asked to return the next day, when they hoped some order would be restored.

By this time May was beyond tears and just wanted to find out what had happened to her family. She went between the hospital and the school several times, and eventually, the next day, she found out the truth. All of the children in her child's class had died. The roof had collapsed completely, crushing them all. Her child was in the morgue, and May identified her. Shortly afterwards, May found her husband at the hospital. He was alive, but his legs had been badly crushed in the earthquake and both had to be amputated below the knee. He remained in hospital for several months, during which time May had been evacuated to live in an encampment outside the town along with many thousands of other people. It looked like a refugee camp. There was barely adequate water for washing, and limited food.

She went to visit her husband every day. He was severely depressed, both by the loss of his legs and the loss of his child. May at this point was psychologically very strong, and helped her husband recover from his injuries. It wasn't until some months later, when her husband was living with her – still in the tent – that she started to have problems. She found herself weeping at random times during the day, and at night had difficulty getting to sleep. She couldn't help thinking about the last moments of her child's life: the terror she must have felt, as the earthquake started and during her last moments as the roof collapsed on them. She wondered if her child had felt a lot of pain before she died or whether it was instant. It was impossible to know, but her mind went over and over the same things.

There was no psychological help available. Even if there had been, there were too many people who needed help. Families comforted each other as best they could. May and her husband struggled. While she went over and over the thoughts about the death of her child, her husband remained depressed and could not or would not talk to her. They lived together yet drifted apart. This went on for months. It was not until over a year later that May had a chance to talk to a psychologist, as we shall see in Chapter 8.

May's example is an extreme case of loss, one that is in some ways impossible to get over. How does one ever recover from the loss of a child? How can someone recover from the loss of both legs, and hence the ability to make a decent livelihood? We shall see later.

The aid worker

This is a very different example, as it does not involve personal loss in the sense of the first case. Chris is an aid worker who has worked with several organizations. Originally from Manchester, he went into aid work after finishing his training as a nurse. He thought he would spend a year or so travelling the world, helping out where necessary, before settling back into a job in England. That was ten years ago. He has spent most of his time in various countries in Africa and Asia, in war zones, post-war zones or famine areas. Sometimes the job is dangerous, sometimes it is boring, but overall Chris has found it very fulfilling. He manages to get home to England once or twice a year for a break and to see his family, and has been happy with that.

Chris has always loved aid work, but a couple of years ago it started to become more difficult. There didn't seem to be any real reason why. The work had not got any more difficult – or it hadn't seemed to. At the time he was working in south Sudan, dealing with refugees from the civil war that had recently ended. Chris found himself getting very tired, and when he went to bed images kept coming into his mind. He tried to shut them out but was never very successful. He found himself sleeping less and less and it started to affect his work. He decided he needed a break and spoke to his manager. The manager was sympathetic and gave Chris a fortnight away in Nairobi, during which Chris spent most of the time drinking, as that was the only way he could get to sleep without the images troubling him. On his return to work he was no better. The symptoms got worse, work became more difficult, and he found it harder to get out of bed in the morning. After another month, he was sent home on sick leave.

When Chris got home to England he went to stay with his family. For the first couple of weeks he did little but sleep and sit around doing very little. His mother was worried about him, but realized that he was over-tired from work. After a couple of weeks, Chris admitted to his mother that he was having problems with thinking about some of the sights that he had seen. He talked it through with her, and in the end started to recover. He felt better for talking things through, and was lucky that his mother was very patient with him.

Eventually Chris could return to work. As you can see, he experienced very different problems from May. He didn't lose anyone, his life wasn't threatened, but he experienced many of the symptoms of traumatic stress: the memories, the problems with sleep, and the way this affected his working life. Traumatic stress is often expressed through physical illness or debility, and can sometimes be difficult to detect. Chris was lucky in having both a manager and a family member who were sympathetic and understood his predicament. Others are not so lucky, and their symptoms may be exacerbated because of people's lack of understanding.

Subclinical distress

As we have seen with the case of Chris, when we talk about post-traumatic stress we are not necessarily talking about a full-blown disorder. It may not be that the person has something we could classify as post-traumatic stress disorder. The National Health Service (NHS) in the UK is now recognizing that with mental health disorders such as PTSD, depression or anxiety, people may experience just some of the symptoms, but this may then later extend to the full disorder. If we can help people at the point where the problems are just starting, then we may be able to stop them getting the full disorder, and so save them and their families a lot of trouble and heartache. The NHS has recently introduced a system whereby people with subclinical problems can be helped by therapists who provide basic forms of therapy or other forms of assistance, such as books like this one.

Someone who has been through a traumatic experience does not, as we have seen, necessarily experience PTSD-related symptoms immediately. These can take months or years to develop. In the meantime, it can be helpful for you to think about what the traumatic event means to you, and how you can make sense of it. This book is intended to help with that process. It is not going to solve all your problems, but it might help ensure that you do not experience the worst forms of PTSD. As we have seen, the symptoms people experience vary a great deal, partly because of the kind of event, with those events that are caused by a person often leading to the worst symptoms, and partly because of the nature of the individual and the way he or she responds to the traumatic event. Our personal characteristics help to determine whether we will experience PTSD after a traumatic event, and this will be the focus of the next chapter.

What we would like you to do before you go any further is to complete some of the questionnaires in Appendix A, specifically the measures of PTSD, anxiety and depression, along with the coping scale. Make a note of your scores. We will ask you to complete them again after you have carried out some of the exercises in the book, with the hope, of course, that your scores will go down. Be honest when you complete the measures; it is only yourself that you are doing this for, and nobody has to see the scores.

3

Personality, coping and support

This chapter looks in more detail at the personal factors that can help determine whether or not we will experience PTSD or other problems after a traumatic event. We will talk about personality factors, the types of coping people use, and social issues such as the support that other people provide. All these are important factors, but none of them alone can predict exactly who will have problems. If we say that PTSD is related to factor X then just because you have a high level of factor X does not mean that you will experience PTSD. None of these factors accurately predict who will have problems; it is much more about the interaction between many factors.

Can I change the way I am?

This has been an argument in psychology ever since it became a discipline back in the nineteenth century. Psychologists have constantly been looking at personality and arguing about whether or not our personalities are fixed or whether they can change. As is usually the case with these kinds of questions, the answer is somewhere in between. We can change some aspects of how we are, but we cannot change others.

Personality

We know that our behaviour is affected by our personalities. There are many ways we can look at personality, but the most common way is known as the Big Five. This is where we look at the main five personality traits:

- Openness to experience (inventive and curious vs. consistent and cautious)
- Conscientiousness (efficient and organized vs. easy-going and careless)

- Extraversion (outgoing and energetic vs. solitary and reserved)
- Agreeableness (friendly and compassionate vs. cold and unkind)
- Neuroticism (sensitive and nervous vs. secure and confident).

(Note that the initial letters spell OCEAN – a good way of remembering them.)

Because these traits are very broad, we cannot on the basis of scores on these characteristics predict who will become traumatized, but in general the higher your score on neuroticism the more likely it is that you may experience PTSD. Similarly, higher scores on the other four traits will predict that you are less likely to experience PTSD. There are a number of versions of the Big Five test. If you are interested, you can find some of these in the internet, but be careful – it is best to use a test that is reliable and valid, and preferably administered by a psychologist. In any case, you can probably estimate whether you are high, medium or low in these five areas compared to people you know. The secret is not knowing your exact score, but being able to think about how you are likely to behave given that you believe yourself to be high in extraversion or low in conscientiousness or whatever. Use the ideas from these personality factors to think about your behaviour.

There are many other personality tests, some of them very detailed and listing 10 or 20 or more personality traits that are said to be able to predict whether or not someone might get a mental illness or be traumatized, and so on. It is best to be wary of many of these. Whatever result you get from them will not tell you whether you will be traumatized or not; there are so many other factors. Let's turn to some of them.

Intelligence

There is some evidence that people who are more intelligent are less likely to be traumatized. This is probably because they are more able to think things through carefully and to make sense of what has happened. We hope that this book will do something similar, in helping to train you to think through your problems and deal with them yourself, rather than having to rely on a therapist or someone else who is an expert in the area. It won't always work, but it often does.

Being a woman

There is a lot of evidence that women are more likely to be traumatized than men after a given event. Of course, this does not mean that women will get traumatized and men will not; it is just about an increased likelihood. There are a number of reasons why women seem to have more problems. The first is a common one found in relation to many mental disorders: women are more likely to report symptoms than men. Women are more likely to go to the doctor and explain the problem. Men tend to avoid the doctor and not tell anyone about their problems and feelings. While this may seem like a good 'tough guy' kind of approach, in the end it can make matters worse. If the man doesn't address the problem, it may build up over time until it is unbearable. Women's apparently greater ability to talk to each other and to doctors about their problems does have advantages!

Coping strategies

This is one of the most important areas to think about when trying to work out the probability of someone having trauma-related problems. There are many theories about coping, but there are some useful ideas about the kinds of coping that work and the kinds of coping that work less well. At the very basic level we all use two forms of coping that we can call processing and avoidance. While we all use both of these, some of us use one more than the other. You should be able to identify your way of responding. When there is a problem, people who tend to use processing will actively think about it and try and find a solution. Those who are avoiders will deliberately avoid thinking about the problem and try to make it disappear.

While the former may look like the most effective way of coping, this is not necessarily the case. Sometimes when we try and think about a problem we go round and round in circles and find it difficult to reach a conclusion. On other occasions, avoiding thinking about a problem can make it go away – especially if there is nothing we can do about it. So both forms of coping can work. It depends on the situation and it depends on the person. Often, we use both together – for instance, if we have an exam coming up we might on one day totally avoid revision and go out with friends (avoidance), while on another day we might sit at the desk and revise (processing). This is normal. After a traumatic event, it is not surprising that we try to use similar coping strategies.

The two sisters

Charlotte and Ann were sisters. They were both in their late teens when their father was killed in an accident. Inevitably it had a profound effect on the family, economically and emotionally. Their mother, who had until then been a housewife, had to go out and find a job. She managed quite well, but the girls responded differently. Ann started going out to pubs and clubs all the time, drinking heavily and having fun. Charlotte wanted to talk about her father all the time, about what he was like, the fun times they had, and even about the details of the accident. Whenever Ann heard Charlotte talk like this, she would get up and leave the room. This went on for some months before Charlotte caught Ann in her room crying. When she asked her what was wrong Ann said nothing, but Charlotte put her arm round her and cuddled her. Ann was silent for a long time and then suddenly started to speak about their father. 'I miss him too, you know,' she said. Charlotte simply nodded. Later in the same week Ann came to Charlotte and asked her about the accident. Up to this point she had refused to hear about it. During the next few weeks they had more conversations and both girls changed. Ann stopped going out so often and getting drunk, and Charlotte started to talk less about her father. The girls had both responded with classic coping strategies: Charlotte used processing and Ann used avoidance.

Processing

Processing helps people to make sense of the traumatic situation, to give it meaning, to develop the narrative. Charlotte talked about the accident because she wanted to make sense of it, she wanted to understand what had happened. Eventually she began to understand, and over time she calmed down. For many people, much of the time, this is the best coping strategy because it helps you resolve your problems. It doesn't work for everyone, but it does for most. Indeed, this book is largely about helping you to use processing even when it is sometimes very difficult to do so. This type of coping is sometimes called 'approach', because the person approaches the problem to deal actively with it.

Avoidance

Ann used avoidance. She didn't want to think about her father's death; it hurt her too much. After a relatively short period of time she stopped using avoidance, because she had reached a point where her level of distress had subsided far enough for her to be ready to talk and understand. There is evidence that people who have been through a traumatic event can use avoidance very effectively for very long periods of time, perhaps permanently, though there is plenty of evidence that avoidance is associated with increased stress, anxiety and depression.

Furthermore, the first author has conducted research with Second World War veterans. This research was conducted 50 years after the end of the war – enough time to 'get over it', you might think. Interestingly, many of the veterans said that they were told to use avoidance after the war – well, they were told to 'forget about it', and their wives were told that if they kept quiet about their husbands' wartime experiences the veterans would soon forget all about them. Many of the veterans said that this avoidance strategy worked for many years. It worked when they got a job, got married and had children. It worked right up until they retired. But then, with the children gone and no work to do, they had a lot more time to think, and they began to think about the war again. At this point many of them started to develop symptoms of war trauma. They started having nightmares; they were getting emotional; they were remembering the people who had died and the incidents where people had died. Some of them found things so difficult that they needed psychological treatment. So while avoidance might work very well, and it might work for decades, there is always the possibility that it may break down as a strategy at some point in the future, and this is why we are recommending that you try and process the information, to deal with the memories so you can think of them without getting too upset. There is also information that stress hormone levels are lower in people who use processing than in those who use avoidance.

Other forms of coping

While there are many measures of coping, one of the most common is the COPE questionnaire developed by Professor Charles S. Carver at the University of Miami. It measures 14 different coping styles, some of which are adaptive, some maladaptive, and many of which can be either adaptive or maladaptive, according to how they are used. You can find a short form of this measure in Appendix A (Measure 5 on p. 109). You should complete and analyse the measure before reading on.

The coping styles measured by the COPE are listed below:

- *Active coping*: taking action and effort to remove or circumvent the stressor (processing, adaptive coping).
- *Planning*: thinking about how to confront the stressor, planning one's active coping efforts (processing, adaptive coping).
- *Use of instrumental support*: seeking assistance, information or advice on what to do (processing, social support, adaptive coping).
- *Use of emotional support*: getting sympathy or emotional support from someone (emotional processing, social support, adaptive coping).
- *Religion*: increased engagement in religious activities (sometimes processing, support, usually adaptive).
- *Positive reframing*: making the best of the situation by growing from it, or viewing it in a more favourable light (processing, adaptive – see Chapter 10).
- *Acceptance*: accepting the fact that the traumatic event has occurred and is real (processing, adaptive).
- *Venting*: of emotions, an increased awareness of one's emotional distress, and a concomitant tendency to ventilate or discharge those feelings (processing, usually adaptive, but can be maladaptive).
- *Denial*: an attempt to reject the reality of the situation (avoidance, maladaptive).
- *Behavioural disengagement*: giving up, or withdrawing effort from, the attempt to attain the goal with which the stressor is interfering (avoidance, maladaptive).
- *Substance use*: turning to the use of alcohol or other drugs as a way of disengaging from the stressor (avoidance, maladaptive).

- *Humour*: making jokes about the stressor (both processing and avoidance, both adaptive and maladaptive).
- *Self-distraction*: psychological self-disengagement away from the goal with which the stressor is interfering through daydreaming, sleep or self-distraction (avoidance, usually maladaptive).
- *Self-blame*: a tendency to blame oneself for either the traumatic event or the negative consequences of the event (maladaptive).

These are the main characteristics of each coping strategy, so you can compare your scores with the list above and see the extent to which you are using adaptive coping strategies. You will also see that some of the strategies are listed as both adaptive and maladaptive. In the extreme, all of them are both adaptive and maladaptive. Trying to process traumatic information, while it is a good thing, can also be damaging to the individual, because you may not be able to deal with the intensity of the emotions associated with that information. There is evidence that people will often use a processing strategy for a period of time until it becomes too difficult, after which they turn to avoidance – basically for a rest from the difficult emotions. Later they will turn back to processing to further deal with the problems.

Another example is that of substance abuse. While of course it is maladaptive to turn to alcohol to deal with problems, as alcohol tends to help one to forget only temporarily (the problem will return in the morning), there is no harm in having a few drinks when it all becomes too much to deal with.

Religion is a complex one. On the one hand, many people make use of religion in their everyday lives both as an explanation for the way the world is and in order to help reduce their stress levels through a form of supernatural social support; on the other hand, trying to explain the world through religion can be seen as a simple way out. With religion one can remove human responsibility from actions (one's own and those of others) and provide a fatalistic explanation or one that absolves the individual from guilt.

As you can see, the interpretations are endless and complex. The final interpretation is yours, and many combinations of these coping strategies can be effective when dealing with traumatic events. Don't worry if your scores seem to be higher for the more maladaptive coping styles: it is important to note that we have conducted research that has shown that these styles can change. One of the first author's PhD students, Saad Jaber, has designed a self help guide aimed at helping people in Baghdad normalize their symptoms and come to terms with their traumatic memories. (Of course, the situation in Baghdad is a complex one, with continual and serious traumatic events, so the need concerns not the *post-*traumatic stress we normally talk about but finding ways of coping with *current* traumatic events.) The guide has been used with large numbers of people, and we have shown that just by reading through it and doing the exercises it contains, people with maladaptive coping strategies have begun to use more adaptive strategies, indicating that styles of coping are not fixed and permanent. Some of the ideas from the guide will be presented at various points in this book.

Help from others (social support)

We all depend on other people – on family and friends, work colleagues and others – to help us through difficult and stressful times. This is never more so than after traumatic events. Research shows that people who think they have good social support are much less likely to experience serious PTSD symptoms. For this reason, it is important to try and make sure such support is available.

The problem is that the symptoms of PTSD include having problems with social relationships. People who are traumatized are often unable to express themselves properly with their friends and relations. It is often the partner who has the most problems, often at several levels. At one level the traumatized person may find it difficult to communicate about the traumatic event, both because it is too difficult to talk about and because of not wanting to upset his or her partner by talking about it. Traumatized people often put a shield around their home, regarding it as a safe place, and so do not talk about what has happened to them to the people in their family. In one way this can be very effective and the traumatized person may feel safer; however, it does not account for the feelings and needs of the family members, who may wish to know more about the traumatic event, and this can make them feel excluded. They may feel the person isn't communicating, and this can cause relationship problems. On the other hand, of course, if all those involved respect this, then it can strengthen the ability of the traumatized person to deal with his or her problems.

Fishing for support

Darren, a 13-year-old boy, had recently witnessed a dreadful car accident. He had been with his best friend Jon when Jon suddenly ran out into the road and was knocked down and instantly killed. Darren saw it all. He saw the accident; he saw the aftermath of the accident. He saw the driver sit rigidly in his car, unable to move because of the shock. He was there, holding Jon's body, when the ambulance men came along and gently took him away. He was at the funeral standing near Jon's parents, listening to them wail.

For a couple of weeks Darren was very quiet. He would sometimes sob to himself, or sit in his room for hours. He had to be kept away from school because he couldn't cope with being there. His mother kept coming to his room, putting her arm around him, talking to him, trying to get him to speak, but it didn't seem to have any effect – in fact Darren would often get angry and run away when his mother tried to speak to him. Nothing seemed to work.

Eventually his father said, 'Let's go fishing.' Darren said nothing, just nodded. It was a Saturday and they went to a quiet stretch of the local river. They sat for most of the day, catching very little and talking very little; but at the end of the day Darren smiled when his dad told him a joke as they were going home. When they got back and Darren had gone upstairs to change, his mother asked his father how it had gone. 'OK. I think I'll take a few days off work and take him again.' He did this and they went fishing on several occasions in the next week. His father didn't say anything about Jon's death, neither did his mother try to talk to him, and eventually it was Darren who brought it up – just a few words now and then. After the week was over Darren said he felt it would be OK to go back to school. Although he took some months to get back to anything like normal, the fishing did seem to make a difference.

This example shows that support does not have to mean talking. Darren's mother meant well in trying to get him to talk, but it was to no avail; he just wasn't ready. His father provided the support he needed just by being there, by showing that he was prepared to take time off work and take him fishing, and not by bothering him with questions.

Another kind of problem that emerges, and that can be linked to the communication issue above, is at the emotional level. You will recall that in the previous chapter we discussed PTSD symptoms and noted that one key symptom is emotional numbing. This occurs – usually at a non-conscious level – because the traumatized person finds it very difficult to deal with the awful emotions associated with the traumatic memory. The fear, the helplessness, the horror – all are difficult to bear, and so the person becomes numbed, becomes unable to feel those emotions. The negative side of this is that it is not only the negative emotions that are numbed: all emotions are numbed, and the person becomes unable to feel the love, joy and happiness associated with the better things in life, the emotions associated with key relationships. If a person cannot feel and express love and happiness – nor appreciate it when it is offered by others – relationships could clearly be affected, possibly causing some real problems.

Perhaps the most difficult problem that can occur between partners is when the traumatized person starts to behave aggressively or violently. This can be quite common, especially in those traumatized by war: where people have been trained in violence, this is considered a normal response to a difficult situation. When a traumatized person starts acting with aggression or violence, with threats or punches, towards a partner, children or other family members, it is very likely that the relationship may be ruined; at the very least it will be severely affected, as the partner and children become frightened whenever the traumatized person is around, and themselves start to behave very differently from normal, treading carefully to avoid the anger.

If you are experiencing these sorts of problems then we suggest that you seek support from an organization such as Relate or one of the other organizations listed in the 'Useful addresses' section at the end of the book.

Of course, these changes that appear in the traumatized person are – often – the result of the traumatic experience, and we would hope that the family members can understand that and act accordingly by providing a lot of support to help the person through this difficult time. That hope is all very well, and there are many people who are strong enough to do this – though few who can put up with their children being beaten – but most of us do not have that strength; most of us cannot put up with such behaviour indefinitely. It is very difficult to deal with the one you love not giving anything positive back, or behaving as though he or she no longer has any love to give.

One thing that can help both partners is having an understanding of what happens – or 'psychoeducation', as it is called. Just being aware that the above can result from the traumatic experience can help both the traumatized person and his or her partner understand, put up with and get past these problems.

Social support does not just come from the person's partner and immediate family: it comes from others, from other relations, from friends and from work colleagues. It also comes from people in the pub, club or wherever the person socializes. These groups provide very different forms of support, and the actual support they provide will depend very much on the traumatized person and his or her individual relationships with them. While, as we have just said, the traumatized person will often protect his or her home as a safe place, there may still be the desire to talk to someone. This may be, for instance, a best friend, a walking companion or someone he or she plays sport with. Often a friend is the one the traumatized person talks to about what has happened and the feelings this has produced. It is easier in many ways because there is both a distance between the two – they don't live together – and a closeness, a bond of friendship, so the friend often understands the other person's strengths and weaknesses very well, and perhaps understands why he or she has responded in this way. For traumatized veterans, the support is often provided by comrades, people who have been through the same things and so understand how they feel. The support can also be provided by formal organizations: for example, The Royal British Legion provides a good form of social support for many former veterans.

Support does not have to be provided by a friend, of course: it can come from anyone. It might be a work colleague, it might be a relation. This isn't the place to tell you who to talk to. You already know.

The other form of social support is provided by people just being around – not people you talk to about your traumatic event and your memories and feelings, but people you are just with, doing the ordinary things in life, whether at work or at leisure. These are the people with whom you can try and get on with your life, with whom you can carry out ordinary tasks that help you keep your world together. However support is used, it is very important for most of us. It is a rare person who does not need the help of others, at least occasionally.

Children's support

A teacher, Sandra, was involved in a car crash where several people were hurt. The crash had been partly her fault and she felt very guilty about it. Her face was quite badly injured and she was in hospital for some weeks, not returning to work until three months after the crash. Sandra taught a class of nine-year-olds, who knew she had been in a crash but didn't know the details. She was dreading what they might say, or that they might taunt her because her face was still a mess.

However, when she walked in on the first day it was to several bunches of flowers and other presents. The class all greeted her positively and it was very clear they were happy to see her back. At the start no one said anything about the state of her face, but eventually, halfway through the morning, one little boy, Tommy, asked her if her face hurt because it looked a mess. There were one or two giggles, but they were quickly stifled. Before Sandra could respond, one of the girls, Vanessa, put her hand up and said, 'Please, Miss, take no notice of Tommy. He is very rude. We are all glad to have you back and teaching us.' Sandra smiled, blinked away her tears and said, 'Thank you, Vanessa, that's good to know.' She turned to Tommy and said, 'Don't worry, Tommy. I bet lots of boys and girls have been wondering about my face.' She then went on to tell them that, yes, it did still hurt a bit, but after another operation it should look normal again. She was pleased this had come out, and now she felt more confident teaching the class. She realized they were her class, the accident didn't matter to them, and they couldn't care less whose fault it was. Young children may often not realize what a support they can be.

Conclusions

In this chapter we have looked at the importance of personality, coping and social support, all things that will help determine how we are going to deal with traumatic events. We are all different, and there is no way we can say that if you have such and such a personality or use such and such a coping style, or have very good support, etc., you either will become traumatized or will not. It is far more complicated than that. What we have tried to do here is to show how these things can be important and how they might interact to help you through your problems. How you might be able to change some of these factors will, we hope, become clearer as you read through the next few chapters.

4

What are the benefits of narrative?

That which does not kill us can only make us stronger.

(Nietzsche)

It is useful, before we go any further, to think about how narrative can not only help reduce the symptoms relating to traumatic stress, but also actually help to make you feel better, even to change you for the better. There is a relatively recent area of psychology called positive psychology, which arose because some people thought – rightly – that there was too much focus on negative aspects of human behaviour. Most applied psychological work had always focused on mental illness, why people are criminals, problems with physical illness, and the difficulties people have at work or with their families. Positive psychology, on the other hand, focuses on those things that are right with the world, or how we can improve our lives. It recognizes that for most of us, most of the time, life is generally pretty good.

While we have looked at how after a traumatic event people may become traumatized, it is also true that – after time – people can benefit from their experience of trauma. We realize that this may be a difficult thing to think about if you have recently experienced such an event, but there is a lot of evidence that the lives of many people change for the better over the longer term. People do start to change the way they think about their lives: how they think about the meaning of life and the meaning of death, and the ways in which they should live their lives and interact with other people. For many, this involves changing jobs or changing the course of their lives, all because of what they have learned by going through the experience of trauma.

The focus on the need for treatment really does bias our perceptions of traumatic events. As we have already said, it is a minority of people who are seriously traumatized by these terrible events.

Nevertheless, these things impact on all of us. For those not seriously affected, it may be relatively easy to deal with the memories of what happened. For those more badly affected, post-traumatic growth can still occur, though you may need extra help from therapists or counsellors (see Chapter 13 for details of the help available from therapists).

This chapter focuses largely on what is known as psychological growth, or how we can grow and develop after traumatic and stressful incidents. It is also about narrative development: how we constantly make meaning from our experiences. As we have already seen, we do not really have any choice about using narrative. It is only in very difficult situations, such as traumatic events, that our ability to develop narratives can fail. It may often take a very long time to rebuild our damaged views about the world, but when we do we are often changed fundamentally. Many people would argue that someone who has lived through a traumatic experience and come to terms with it is in some way a better person, someone who has a greater understanding of the world precisely because of those experiences. Many people go on to help others with similar problems by starting self-help groups or talking to others about their experiences. In this way they are finding new meaning in their lives by supporting others.

What is positive psychology?

While positive psychology may be relatively recent within the discipline of psychology, the ideas behind it have been with us for thousands of years. We can explore philosophy, literature and religion to see where the ideas come from. Buddhism is concerned with the attempt to come to terms with human suffering. Buddha was the enlightened teacher who understood a great deal about human life and suffering and who tried to show the way out of the cycle of suffering and rebirth and the achievement of Nirvana. Buddhist teachings focus on the development of mindfulness and meditation and how these can help you rid yourself of suffering. Mindfulness has become a part of mainstream psychology and is designed to help alleviate problems such as post-traumatic stress.

Within the Christian tradition, the suffering of Jesus is seen as a metaphor for a means of saving other people from suffering. This is a common theme in many religions. One of the purposes of religion is to provide an organized way of explaining how and why people suffer in the world and the means by which this suffering can be alleviated. While for many people religion serves little purpose, for some this is one of the key means of understanding why they suffer and of finding a way – through their god – to reduce that suffering, as the religion itself provides the explanation for the problems people have.

Shakespearean tragedy, as described in *Othello*, *Macbeth*, *Hamlet* and *King Lear*, is a representation of how traumatic events resolve themselves. As Shakespearean tragedies are designed to provide entertainment over and above an explanation for suffering, the plays do not end well for the main protagonists, but we can draw from these plays a sense of meaning-making, a sense of how narratives develop. All tragedies, not just Shakespearean ones, have a number of stages. These include:

- the precipitant: an act of shame or horror, in our case the traumatic event;
- suffering: which is only tragic if it provides some insight or understanding;
- knowledge: about the world, which is derived from the insight into the suffering;
- affirmation: that life is worthwhile, the dignity of the human spirit.

These relate well to our ideas about how narrative is important for meaning-making and the resolution of traumatic memories, and show how these ideas have been with us for centuries. In recent years, evidence has accumulated about the importance of these stages of tragedy in relation to traumatic events such as chronic illness, heart attacks, breast cancer, HIV, rape and combat. While Shakespeare may have been telling stories, they were based on genuine ways of dealing with the world, which is why these stories have been so successful. We understand what they mean.

Positive psychology

The role of positive psychology is – unlike much of traditional psychology – to understand something about the more positive aspects of human life, and to encourage these in people. It focuses on positive experiences, positive traits and positive institutions. According to Martin Seligman, the psychologist who introduced positive psychology, the usual focus on pathology was an approach that lacked the positive features which make life worthwhile, such as hope, wisdom, creativity, futuremindedness, courage, spirituality, responsibility and perseverance – all areas that are usually ignored within psychology or are seen as transformations of negative aspects such as mental illness.

Growth

There are many terms that have been used by psychologists and others to describe post-traumatic growth, including 'stress-related growth', 'perceived benefits', 'adversarial growth', 'thriving', 'blessings', 'by-products' and 'positive readjustment'. Basically, the idea of growth, whatever we choose to call it, is concerned with how after a traumatic event – admittedly often a long time after a traumatic event – people feel that in some way the experience of trauma has led to some positive change in their understanding of life. It might be that they feel they have a better understanding of the meaning of death, or perhaps the fragility of life, and this then leads to changes in behaviour, perhaps respecting people more or making the most of life instead of frittering it away. It is not possible to say exactly what those positive changes will be, but to the person who has experienced growth there is a sense of a better understanding of oneself, other people and perhaps the world.

Existential change

Another way of putting these changes is to talk of existential change. Jean-Paul Sartre's existentialist philosophy declared that the meaning of life was developed by the individual: unless a person decided for him or herself what life was all about, it was little more than simple existence. The notion of existential change is important for post-traumatic growth. The traumatic memories are resolved through such change: that is, growth is related to the meaning you put on life. This means that there are certain stages: the traumatic event itself, the initial negative responses (fear, anxiety, traumatic memories), the search for meaning to make sense of the trauma and loss, and finally the attainment of meaning. It is not until some meaning or sense is made of the traumatic event that post-traumatic growth can occur. This growth can mean a fundamental change of identity, with the person thinking of him or herself as someone totally different from the person before the traumatic event.

Clearly this can have serious consequences for someone's life, in terms of relationships with family and friends, work and life generally. It is not uncommon for marriages to split after a traumatic event, both at the stage of the initial response to the trauma, when life becomes difficult for everyone around the traumatized person, and also at the stage of growth, when the traumatized person is – in effect – becoming a new person. That new person may not be compatible with the old one, and relationships can suffer.

What appears to happen, then, with growth is that identity can change, and through this the person develops a greater sense of autonomy and control over the world, which is related to a perceived greater understanding of the world. This happens at the personal and social level, and it is easy to see how it relates to ideas from philosophy and religion regarding the nature of suffering and recovery from suffering.

There are many examples of people around the world who have worked at the social and community level, drawing on their own traumatic experiences to grow psychologically through helping others. Examples include: Diana Lamplugh, the mother of a murdered young woman, who set up the Suzy Lamplugh Trust to help other women; Nelson Mandela and the way he brought the people of South Africa together after the collective trauma of apartheid; Leonard Cheshire, who set up homes for the disabled after his experiences as a pilot in the Second World War. There are numerous other examples, some well known, others less so.

Measuring growth

What we do not know is what proportion of people experience growth. Previous research has shown anything from only 3 per cent for people who have been bereaved through to 98 per cent in one study of breast cancer. These are extremes. It is likely that the very high percentage for breast cancer was because the people involved were those who had survived the disease, and so had hope for the future. The other problem is that the concept of growth is not very well defined, so people are measuring different things. That can be seen by the number of different questionnaires that are used to measure growth. Some names include: the Post-traumatic Growth Inventory, the Stress-related Growth Scale, the Changes in Outlook Questionnaire, the Thriving Scale, the Illness Cognition Questionnaire, the Perceived Benefits Scale and the Psychological Well-being–Post-traumatic Changes Questionnaire. While all these are measuring post-traumatic growth, they are not all measuring it in the same way.

A good recent example is the Psychological Well-being–Post-traumatic Changes Questionnaire (PWB–PTCQ) developed by the psychologists Stephen Joseph and Steve Regel. While the name doesn't trip off the tongue, the measure is a good one, focusing on one's personal *psychological* well-being. It measures several characteristics of psychological well-being, as shown in Table 4.1.

Table 4.1 Characteristics of psychological well-being

Characteristic	What this means
Autonomy	You are self-determining, and can resist social pressures to think and act in certain ways
Environmental mastery	You have a sense of control and can make effective use of opportunities
Positive relations with others	You have warm, satisfying and trusting relationships with other people and you are capable of empathy, affection and intimacy
Personal growth	You have a feeling of continued development and you are open to new experiences
Purpose in life	You have clear goals in life and have beliefs about life having a purpose
Self-acceptance	You have a positive attitude towards yourself and feel positive about your life

You can find a copy of this questionnaire in Appendix A, along with instructions on how to score it (Measure 6, p. 111). It is likely that you will score higher in certain categories than others. Do not worry if this is the case; it is perfectly normal. Also, if you have recently experienced a traumatic event you may score quite low on the scale. Growth often comes after a hard battle with the effects of trauma, though growth can be experienced at the same time as symptoms of traumatic stress. You should use this measure occasionally over time to see if you are experiencing any changes.

What are the personal factors that relate to growth?

There are a number of factors that seem to be related to growth. These relate to how we interact with the world. One unusual finding is that those people who are most likely to report a higher level of threat and danger in a traumatic situation are also more likely to report experiencing growth. While at one level this looks unlikely, it is probably found because those of us who think more about the traumatizing situation – i.e. who perceive a greater level of threat – are perhaps the same people who are then able to think about it differently – and more positively – over time. There is also evidence that women are more likely to experience growth. Again, this is probably linked to women being more likely to both think about and report higher levels of stress and growth. There is a level of openness in many women that we don't find in so many men. Other factors that predict growth include being younger – is it more difficult for older people to come to terms with trauma? – and being more highly educated or earning more money. Perhaps these relate to cognitive ability.

Personality is also related to growth. Of the Big Five personality factors, four are positively related to growth, and one is more related to post-traumatic stress disorder. The four factors relating to growth include higher levels of extraversion, openness to experience, agreeableness and conscientiousness. Neuroticism is correlated with PTSD. Other personality variables that relate to growth include higher self-esteem and optimism.

People who are good at coping are more likely to experience growth, whether they focus on coping by thinking through the problem (what psychologists call cognitive processing) or by focusing on dealing with the emotions. Whichever is used (and most of us use both), growth is associated with the effectiveness of the coping style rather than the coping style itself. Growth is also linked to effective social support, so those who see themselves as having good social support are often the ones who experience most growth.

The problem with this is that it doesn't apply to everyone. Psychological research is equivocal. The above is true for many people but not for everyone. Furthermore, people's personality and coping styles can change over time and with practice. This is another reason why we are recommending a narrative approach, as alongside the development of narrative a person does learn to cope more effectively.

Disrupted narratives and post-traumatic growth

We have already shown that after a traumatic event there can be a total destruction of the narratives we have about ourselves, other people, and the world. We can, however, then rebuild our narratives and in the end experience post-traumatic growth. An example of this was described by the American psychologist Robert Neimeyer and relates to a woman called Sarah.

Sarah's story
Sarah was getting her children ready for school one morning when she received a long-distance telephone call. She could not at first make out who it was, but then realized it was her brother, who sounded very panicky. He told her to turn on the television, which she did, and then she saw the twin towers of the World Trade Center in New York burning. Her brother worked in one of the towers. He wanted her to tell him what was happening in the very offices where he worked – and where he had reported for work an hour before. When she saw the pictures, Sarah felt a wave of terror passing through her, as the flames and smoke were just a few floors above where her brother was working. She could hear screams in the background on the phone. For the next 22 minutes Sarah encouraged her brother to make his way down the smoke-filled staircase towards safety. The horror became much worse when she saw the images of the collapsing structure, just as her brother reached the eleventh floor. At that moment she heard a roar in the receiver and the

phone went dead. She knew that she had just watched and heard the moment her brother died.

Over the next few months Sarah was flooded with imagery of the burning and collapsing buildings. This was made worse by the intrusive memories of the people grieving their dead. She found herself, both during the day and in her dreams at night, picturing her brother's last half-hour trying to get down the stairs. She obsessively tried to piece together the fragments from her memories of the phone call and the information from media reports. She struggled with her previous optimistic narratives about the world being a safe place, life being predictable and the universe just. Now she felt that this whole structure was destroyed.

Sarah had a complicated grief reaction, but this destruction of her world view led to processes of narrative revision, and over time – and using therapy – she managed to slowly rebuild a more coherent account of the traumatic imagery and put this in place among her larger narratives about the world. This finally led Sarah to a more complex world view which acknowledged the reality of death, the preciousness of life and how humans were at the same time resilient and vulnerable. What happened was that in the end Sarah managed to experience post-traumatic growth via the struggle to get past the traumatic disorganization of her life narratives after the tragic loss of her brother.

Post-traumatic growth and therapy

We will be talking more about therapy later on, but it is worth noting that while much therapy is about the reduction of symptoms, it can be made more effective by incorporating ideas about post-traumatic growth. Many therapies can make use of these ideas, particularly those that explicitly use narrative methods but also more standard therapies such as cognitive behavioural therapy. We will be talking about how you can make use of therapeutic journals, expressive writing and oral methods in the next few chapters, and when you are looking at these methods keep the idea of growth in your mind. Narrative methods and post-traumatic growth work well together.

Conclusion

Post-traumatic growth is an important subject when we are thinking about how people deal with traumatic stress. Post-traumatic growth is about more than just non-negative thinking: it is about profound positive change that results from dealing well with the problems life can throw at you. It is about making sense of the world. It is about psychological well-being, health and positive relationships. What is interesting is that post-traumatic stress disorder and post-traumatic growth are not the opposite ends of a continuum, as there is ample evidence that people can experience both post-traumatic stress and post-traumatic growth at the same time. As complex creatures, people who are traumatized are constantly trying to deal with their memories, beliefs and feelings, and so even though they may still experience symptoms, they can at the same time have an awareness of the more positive aspects of life. It is worth bearing in mind that growth is not – except in psychology – a new idea. It has been around for thousands of years, throughout human history, and so it is perfectly natural for people affected by difficulties in life to think about the positive things that have resulted from their difficulties.

5

The stories we tell

As we noted in the Introduction, we are all storytellers. We can't help it; it is what makes us human. We tell stories in every situation we are in. If we are not telling stories we are listening to stories. We are involved in stories. It is one of the main ways in which we make sense of the world. This is a bold claim, but just think about it: think about the situations where we are using stories – however simple – and where we are not using stories.

Here are a few examples of stories. The obvious ones include reading a book, a magazine or a newspaper. Journalists use stories to tell us about events in the world. Every class a teacher has with pupils is telling a story, whether it is a story about history, geography, mathematics . . . When people are talking to their friends about what they have done during the day they are telling them a story. Many people keep diaries, accounts of what they have done and their interpretations of what has happened (without the interpretation it is pure description, and we wouldn't call it a story).

Epic storytelling

We know about the so-called oral traditions in many societies, particularly those without writing, where the great stories of the tribe are told by special storytellers who are responsible for handing down the knowledge of the tribe. They learn the stories and then tell them to the younger members of the tribe, some of whom then themselves become storytellers, weaving new information about what has happened into the stories of events from the more distant past. In many ways we in the modern world have lost our ability to tell – and listen to – such epic stories, because we now rely on books, teachers and the internet to store our knowledge; perhaps we rely on them too much. Perhaps TV soap operas are modern epics in the way they deal with human drama and traumatic events; even if they are somewhat absurd and exaggerated for tragic effect, they are popular culture dealing with the real stories of life.

What makes a story?

When is something not a story? A story should include certain key characteristics:

- There should be a sense of time; there is a chronological order with each event logically following another.
- There should be a sense of structure, with a beginning, a middle and an end.
- A story needs a sense of coherence, where the listener can make sense of the story as a whole; it threads together; there are no missing links.
- There should be one or more points of view, so there is an interpretation by the person giving the story. Perhaps this person puts across other people's points of view too, so there can be a debate or argument.
- There is an audience, whether they are real or imagined, whether they are present when the story is told or not.
- There is interpretation; it is not just a descriptive account.
- A story can be fictional, partly fictional or factual.
- A story can be oral, written or artistic.

You can probably think of other elements of a story, but these are the main ones.

There are some key differences between stories depending on how they are being told and to whom, and some of these are important for our purposes. For instance, there is a big difference between writing a story for an imaginary audience and telling a story to someone who is present. If you are writing a story you have to think about what needs to be said and how it needs to be said as you are writing it. There won't normally be an opportunity to adapt it once the person is reading it. If, on the other hand, you are telling your story verbally you can adapt it in accordance with how the other person responds to what you say. If you say something he or she doesn't understand you can repeat it in different words; if there are elements the person would like you to elaborate on you can do this; if there are parts the person doesn't want to hear you can keep quiet about these things. A story told orally to a person who is present is developed through the interaction with the person. It is not usually a monologue. This is important for our purposes.

Problems with stories and the need for an audience

There are many occasions when we – usually the audience, but sometimes the storyteller – do not understand the story, when the storyline isn't clear or has not been thoroughly developed. As mentioned above, if we simply describe something without interpretation then we don't have a story. If something does not make sense in terms of a beginning, a middle and an end we don't have a story. If there is just a simple list of items there is no story. For instance, a shopping list with bacon, milk, eggs, tea and bread on it doesn't make any sense of a story, but if a person is inviting someone to stay over for the night and is going to cook breakfast in the morning then we start to get the elements of a story. Then an audience might become intrigued about who was coming over to stay and why, so the storyteller would have to develop the story further. This illustrates the importance of the audience in story development – the need for motivation to create a sensible story.

Autobiography

The biggest story we have in our lives is the story about our life, our own autobiography. This is a very complex story, and one that is told (and withheld) in different ways according to our audience. If we are telling our children the story of our lives we may tell it in a way that withholds certain pieces of information and emphasizes others. We may tell a slightly different story to our partner, and yet another to our friends or our work colleagues. They are all variations on the same story, but we may want some people to know some elements and others to know something different. It is about the way we want to project ourselves; whether it is 'warts and all' will depend on who we are talking to. Most of us, most of the time, also want to portray a positive image of our lives, so we may omit or downplay some of the mistakes we have made. Of course, people with conditions such as depression may emphasize the negative aspects of life in order to show themselves and others what a terrible life they have led. The problem with traumatized people is that it becomes very difficult for them to tell the story of their life, because it is broken, fragmented and doesn't make sense to them, let alone tell a coherent story to others.

Sharing the story

It is up to you whether you wish to share your trauma story with other people, or perhaps with a single special person. While most narratives are created for sharing with an audience, some of our personal narratives can remain just that – personal and private. On the other hand, many people who have been traumatized want to share their story, their experiences, with others, as it gives them a sense of being unburdened: the weight of the traumatic experience is lifted by the sharing of that experience. There is often also an educational element; traumatized people want to share their experiences, and what they have learned from them, with others, so that these others may not have to go through what they have been through.

How can that story be shared? Again, that is a personal preference. It is important, however, that the person who is being told the story actually wants to hear it. Many people find it difficult to hear about other people's traumatic experiences, and this can commonly be the case for close family members. In Chapter 3 we discussed social support, and it is important to reiterate that, for some people, the home is a place that is safe from trauma. It may be that sharing memories and thoughts with someone who lives in the same house may itself damage the relationship. Telling a loved one about terrible thoughts and experiences can be damaging to that loved one, and to oneself.

6

Before you start the exercises

Dealing with traumatic memories is difficult. That is their nature. They are extremely distressing and cause a range of emotions, from anger and fear to helplessness and horror. Depending on what actually happened there can be feelings of shame or of guilt. The whole gamut of – mainly – negative emotions applies to traumatic memories. If you are traumatized then the memories can be difficult or impossible to deal with; however, if you have got to the stage of reading this book, you have already started on the road to recovery. No one should claim that it is easy. A traumatized person is seldom 'cured' in the sense of going back to being the same person he or she was before the traumatic experience. Such experiences change us for ever. That does not mean, though, that the change has to remain negative. We have already seen how many people learn to cope with their memories, and often experience psychological growth.

The problem with traumatic memories is the link between the memory and the emotion. It is a very strong link in that it is very difficult to think of the memory without experiencing the emotion. The aim of recovery is to find a way of removing the link so that you can think of the memory without necessarily experiencing the intense emotion. The role of the narrative is to help you in that process, to help you make sense of what happened, to understand it, so that you don't feel those emotions – or at least don't feel them so intensely.

Warning

All of the techniques we describe may cause you to feel very distressed and emotional. Before you undergo any of them, make sure you are in the right frame of mind to do so. If you do experience serious distress and feel that you cannot deal with it, go and visit your GP and explain your situation. Your GP may then advise you to seek help from a professional therapist or counsellor.

Relaxation

You can learn to control your trauma-related distress by teaching yourself to relax. There are good techniques that we all use, such as walking the dog, going for a walk in the countryside, having a bath or listening to relaxing music. These may work for you in relation to many of the normal stressors of life, but they may not work in relation to traumatic stress. This kind of intense distress is more difficult to deal with, but it is manageable.

When you use the writing techniques we describe, you are likely to experience distress. You might feel distress as you are writing, or you might feel anxious when you know you are going to write. There are some relatively simple relaxation techniques you can learn that should help you ease that distress. It is important that you practise these techniques before you attempt the exercises, so they are easier to do.

General relaxation

- Find a quiet place where you will not be disturbed. Sit or lie down comfortably.
- Think about your body: are there areas where you are tense? Do some simple stretching exercises to remove the tension.
- Concentrate on your breathing. Breathe deeply, gently and regularly.
- Tense and then relax each part of your body in turn, starting with your feet and working your way up to your head.
- As you do this, think of warmth and heaviness in each part.
- Try to push any distracting thoughts out of your head.
- When you have released the tension from your body and pushed distracting thoughts out of your head, sit like this, with your eyes closed, for about 20 minutes. At the end of this time, take a few deep breaths, open your eyes and sit/lie still for a few moments, and then get up.
- Try to do this on a regular basis.

Talking to a friend

While you may not want to share your traumatic memories with people, just talking to them about the ways they relax can help.

Using the internet

There is a lot of advice about relaxation techniques on the internet. A few sites are listed at the end of the book, but there are many more.

Going to a class

Ask your GP about local relaxation classes.

Buying a CD

Materials about relaxation are widely available; some come with relaxing music.

Thinking about your safety

Some of these exercises will make you think quite deeply about the traumatic experience. You need to be sure that you can handle that. In the first place, if you are very badly affected by these experiences then you should consider seeing a therapist. We discuss therapy in Chapter 13. A therapist or counsellor can provide a safe environment for you to discuss your thoughts and feelings about the traumatic event. As we have already discussed, we often depend on other people for support, and you need to think about whether you need the support of a therapist, or whether you get enough support from your friends and family. Perhaps you do get support from the latter. If so, will they still be able to provide this support if you start going through some of the exercises in this book and find yourself thinking more about the traumatic event? If you get angry, will you be supported? If you find you can't go into work, will your boss and your colleagues support you? Think seriously about these things before doing the exercises.

On the positive side, there is good evidence that doing these narrative exercises can have quite a fast positive effect. They are designed to help you make sense of your experiences quickly, using mind processes that we all use every day. You do not have to learn any new skills, just develop the ones you already have for the context of the traumatic event.

Dealing with your traumatic thoughts will entail experiencing intense emotions. You need to be able to manage these. There are many ways of doing this, including learning relaxation exercises, talking to a trusted friend or relation, or going for a walk (as discussed in the next chapter). Depending on the experience, you may also have a sense of loss and a need to grieve. Do not worry about this; it is normal to go through a grieving process. The main thing to try and focus on is the future: you are working through your traumatic memories in order to have a happier and more settled life. Try to keep your focus on this, and on how it will be better not only for yourself but for those around you, your family and friends, once you feel better. It will be difficult and it may take time, but it will be worth it.

Writing, thinking, talking

The exercises in the next few chapters are about creating narratives in a number of ways, mainly writing, thinking or talking (but also art and drama). Many people write about their traumatic experiences completely sure that they are never going to show them to anyone else. Sometimes people write about their experiences and then tear up or burn the pages. This is quite common, particularly if you are feeling vulnerable, and think that if other people saw what you have written you would be somehow weakened. In these cases, this is still a narrative, but with you as the audience. This is writing for oneself, to make sense of whatever it is you are writing about. A Second World War veteran said that although he wasn't generally troubled by his memories of the war there were occasions when he was reminded of something unpleasant, and in order to work through the memory he would take a blank sheet of paper and a pen and sit and write a poem. There was no intention of publishing the poems or of showing them to anyone else, but the actual act of writing, structured writing, helped him to resolve his traumatic memory, to make sense of it, by writing to himself.

Many people do not like writing, and for them it is sometimes better to think the problem through, working out what it is and coming up with a solution, going through it in the mind until it makes sense.

After writing and thinking there is talking, and many of us talk to friends and relations about our problems. As we have already said, many traumatized people do not, for good reasons, want to talk to their closest relatives (often their partner) because they want to retain the idea of home as a safe place; but they may well want to talk to a friend, to use the friend to share ideas, to bounce them around, to make sense of them.

So we have three straightforward ways of doing stories: writing, thinking and talking. There is nothing profound in this; it is what we all do, every day. Some of us choose one method, some another. Many of us make use of all three at different times. When the problem is a relatively straightforward one, we do this automatically. There is a slight disruption to our thinking and we can relatively simply resolve the problem. It is nothing special, just the way that human minds work.

Children

Children are a special group when it comes to traumatic stress. While they are no more or less resilient than adults, they may need special help as – especially with young children – it may be difficult to predict how they may respond to their traumatic experiences. The exercises in this book are not specifically written for children, though some are suitable and some have been used with children, such as the expressive writing tasks and art and drama therapy. We do not recommend that young children undertake these tasks because there is the problem of knowing how they will respond to their traumatic experiences. Young children often do not verbalize their problems but can be encouraged to act them out with dolls, puppets or art. These techniques, used with children, should be conducted by a specialist.

Guided Narrative Techniques (GNTs)

We will now turn to the exercises. We call these Guided Narrative Techniques because that is what they are. We all use narratives every day but sometimes, as in the traumatic situation, we find them very difficult to create, so what follows is simply a series of exercises that provide you with guidance to develop your own narratives. The table in Appendix B illustrates at a glance the kinds of activities involved in each of these GNTs.

7

Walking and talking, walking and thinking

There is evidence that there are significant benefits to walking. Physically, these include general increased fitness and fewer weight-related problems, lower blood pressure, less joint pressure and lower likelihood of a stroke. People also feel generally more energetic. Mentally, walking improves sleep, and can lighten mood in depressed people. Walking itself can act as a kind of meditation. A walk somewhere nice can help you focus on the environment rather than on what is wrong with you. People will often talk about the value of walking in the sense of it enabling you to focus on elements of your body or your breathing. So the benefits of walking are complex: the more you walk, the fitter you feel, the happier you feel and the higher your self-esteem, and in the end it can also benefit diet and nutrition. It is one of those rare activities that do not have any drawbacks.

Walking, for the traumatized person, has several benefits. In the first place, walking means you get out of the house. Sitting in the same place every day has severe drawbacks: it encourages rumination, just going over and over the same thoughts in your head; it encourages a bad diet and a lack of fitness; you are less likely to see friends. Linked to this is the way in which walking is relaxing. The easy repetitive physical activity not only improves fitness, it improves mood.

For our purposes, the main benefit of walking is the way it helps you think. Walking is one of the best ways of working out solutions to your problems, whether you are walking alone and thinking or walking with someone else and talking. While we do not understand the actual mechanisms, walking gives you the capacity to think more clearly.

Walking is our most natural form of exercise. When walking we do not have to think about the mechanics involved, yet the act itself does somehow enhance our ability to think. Walking jogs the mind into activity. Many people will claim that they have their best thoughts and ideas while out walking, and that walking enables them to think things through. Here we are not distinguishing between walking alone and thinking and walking with a friend and talking and thinking. Both activities are enhanced by the walk.

Of course, not everyone likes to go for a walk, and not everyone has somewhere nice to walk; the maimed veteran who has lost his legs is likely to feel depressed and angry when he thinks about walking. But this does not – except in extreme cases of paralysis or amputation – stop people from taking some form of physical exercise. Some people gain a lot from jogging or running or playing sports. The physical stimulation generally makes people feel both physically and mentally better. Physical exercise leads to increased fitness, and increased fitness is associated with psychological well-being and mental alertness.

Exercises for walking and talking/thinking

For some people it is enough to let their minds wander: during that meandering, problems relating to either everyday life or the traumatic event can be at least partially resolved. For most of us, however, this is not the case. Just as we need exercise to get physically fit, so we need mental stimulation to get mentally fit. If you have problems with traumatic memories, they are not going to go away without at least some careful thinking.

A good starting point

A good starting point is to try and think about what is troubling you. Go into as much detail as you can. This applies whether you are walking alone or walking with a friend.

What is it about the traumatic event that bothers you?

- Is it a particular memory of something that happened?
- Is it a memory of something that a person (or you) did or didn't do?
- How do you feel when you think about this memory? Do you feel angry, sad, depressed, fearful or anxious?

- Does it make you want to do something, e.g. hit out at someone, stay in your room, cry?
- Do you feel guilty or ashamed about something you should or should not have done?
- Does the memory make you feel differently about other people, e.g. your wife or husband, other family members, other people generally? In what ways? Are you less loving, more careless? Are you aggressive?
- Have your thoughts and feelings changed since the traumatic event? What has changed and how?

When do your traumatic memories bother you?

- At night in bed (perhaps as bad dreams, or when you are unable to sleep)?
- When you are with particular people, e.g. someone who was also involved?
- When you are in a particular situation, e.g. where the event happened or drinking in a pub?

What do you usually do when you think about this memory?

- Something negative, such as getting angry at someone, lashing out, drinking alcohol, taking drugs, hiding away?
- Something more positive, such as trying to control your thoughts and feelings, or going for a walk on your own?

Overall, what are the important ways in which the traumatic event has changed your life?

- Do you see yourself as in some ways a worse person, e.g. towards others at work or in your social life?

Once you have given a lot of thought to the questions above, and perhaps discussed them with a trusted friend, you may find that just this process of thinking has helped you understand yourself better, and that you have a clearer idea of how you have changed since the traumatic event, both within yourself and in your dealings with other people. You may find yourself understanding the problem better and perhaps thinking about how to solve it – something which will create further questions for you to answer, particularly about why you are having problems with memories, thoughts and feelings. You now need to think about how these problems can be resolved. This is not necessarily straightforward and may involve tackling a number of issues separately. Before that, you may need to control the anxiety linked to your thoughts and feelings.

Controlling your thoughts and feelings

If you have a problem with anxiety, begin by thinking about how to calm yourself down. This might be as simple as taking a series of slow deep breaths, concentrating on the breathing itself rather than the thoughts that might be going through your mind. Alternatively it might involve a simple technique such as pushing your thumb into your forefinger; this is something that you can do without anyone noticing, but if you train yourself to relax when you feel your thumb pressing against your forefinger it can work well.

Can you learn to control your feelings? Part of this is relaxation, as described above, but part of it is also thinking about why you have these feelings and trying to dismiss the negative ones – the ones that make you feel bad – and replace them with more positive feelings. This can be very difficult, but that is the point of the walk. The repetitive exercise of moving your arms and legs calms the mind and helps you concentrate. If you can take a walk in the countryside, do so; it is more tranquil and hence more beneficial. As you walk admire the environment, the trees, the scenery. Smell the fresh air. Look at the animals and the insects. If you can get into the right frame of mind, calm and peaceful, it will make it easier to actively think about your problems. If you cannot get out into the countryside you can still walk and observe. Look at the fine buildings and think about the people who built them. Walk in the parks and observe nature. Try to find somewhere quiet.

Learning from walking can be difficult. It is not easy to calm down and relax when you have terrible traumatic memories that are bothering you. It may take practice and it may take time. Try to be patient. Make a habit of walking every day if possible, and actively think about what we are saying here. There is no guarantee it will work, but it certainly won't work without effort.

At the very least, through walking you are getting exercise and learning to control your feelings.

Dealing with negative or distorted beliefs

Let us turn to what you think about yourself, other people and the world in relation to the traumatic event. Psychologists often call these 'distorted' beliefs because they distort your view of the world. They make you think badly about yourself and others, and make it difficult to get on with things as you used to. Once you have been able to control your feelings using your walks, you can try and think about how you might control your thoughts and beliefs. Thoughts are not separate from feelings; you feel the way you do because you think the way you do, and vice versa, but in order to be able really to concentrate on your beliefs you do need to have some control over your feelings.

It is important to try and replace negative beliefs with 'better' beliefs (if that is the right word). For instance, if you feel that you did not behave well in the traumatic situation, try to work out why. Work out what you could have done instead. Don't think about being a hero. Most of us are not heroes. Just learn to accept that what you did is what you did and nothing can be changed – except the way you think about it. In many cases there will have been nothing else you could reasonably have done, but even if there had been, this was a life-threatening and/or frightening situation and no one would expect you to have behaved differently. You could reason that you would behave differently next time – but don't spend too much time fantasizing about heroics. We are all normal human beings with normal skills and normal failings.

If the problem was the behaviour of another person, e.g. a rape or a shooting, try not to judge all people by that individual. Whatever you might be thinking at the moment, however much you may despise or fear other people, most of us are perfectly normal, reasonably good people who generally try to get along with others and do so most of the time. Train yourself to think like that. Look at the evidence. Look at how most people are generally good and try not to have a distorted negative belief about others. Again, this takes time and effort, but it is worth it.

Conclusion

We started this chapter by talking about the nature of storytelling, and then going through the process of how you can develop your own stories through 'walking and talking': that is, moving from a position where the memories of the trauma are fragmented, the feelings are difficult to cope with, and thoughts about the self, other people and the world are negative or distorted. By effective use of walking and talking the traumatized person can create a more or less sophisticated story about the traumatic event and make sense of it. Stories nearly always have an intended audience but it is of less importance whether this story is actually told to other people. In the end, though, many of us feel unburdened when we are able to talk to someone about our experiences.

In Chapter 4 we talked about the idea of post-traumatic growth, of how you can grow mentally from traumatic experiences. The beginning of growth is about changing the way you think about the world, and from there you can develop a wiser and personal understanding of the meaning of life and death. We hope that you may begin to experience something positive after practically applying this chapter. It may then be worth completing the measures again and seeing what has changed. Hopefully, your scores on PTSD, anxiety and depression may have reduced and your score on growth increased, but don't worry if they haven't: the exercises we have in later chapters may be more appropriate for you personally, and we will provide more detailed guidance about how to express yourself and more help on how to change.

This chapter has begun to explore how we can develop our own narratives, either alone or with a little help from others. Walking and talking is fine for some people, those who can still make effective use of narrative. Often, though, it is not possible to work it through by yourself, just by thinking about it. The next chapter focuses on providing some more structured guidelines for the development of narratives.

8

Guided writing techniques

I live in the present and with the passage of time most of the experiences I have been through have grown unreal and faint. Yet the urge to recall them in writing has persisted. I think that the reason for this is that I have never been able to believe that anything had really and thoroughly happened to me until I had written it down . . . For writing a thing down means ordering it and arranging it. The letter writer or autobiographer takes the chaotic material he finds in his memory and organizes it, eliminating what is trivial and thus allowing what is significant to stand out.

(Gerald Brenan, *Personal Record 1920–1972*.
Jonathan Cape, 1974)

We have discussed how narratives can be developed through a number of different approaches. In the previous chapter we focused on the technique of walking and talking/thinking. In this chapter we focus on a slightly different approach, that of writing about whatever it is that is upsetting. Again, this is something people have done for many years – whether they have intended to write just for themselves in a diary or journal or whether they have written articles, pamphlets or books for publication, it amounts to the same thing. Meaning-making through the written word is – or can be – as effective as meaning-making through storytelling.

Abreaction

Therapists and researchers have used writing as a therapeutic tool for many years. Carl Jung, an early psychotherapist who originally worked with Sigmund Freud before they had a dispute about psychoanalysis, suggested the concept of 'abreaction', which means living through or reliving a traumatic event so that the emotions linked to that event are re-experienced and thus become more manageable. Jung was writing at a time when most people thought that if a person was traumatized the best thing would be to forget all about it. He realized that people didn't forget so easily, and that the best way of dealing with the emotions was to confront them.

Abreaction derived from psychoanalytic notions about the concept of unconsciousness. Jung and others thought that trauma-related emotions are stored deep in the mind, in the unconscious, and that reminders might bring them back into consciousness. Nowadays psychoanalysis is not very popular among mainstream therapists, but it doesn't matter what we call it: we know that if people write about their difficult emotions, then for many those emotions will become less of a problem. We are concerned with the practical benefits, not the theory.

In the 1970s, Jamie Pennebaker of the University of Texas started working on what he called 'expressive writing'. His initial experiments involved getting students to write for 15–20 minutes a day, on four consecutive days. The students were told either to write about a personal trauma or stressful event or to write about something trivial. The former group were asked to discuss the emotions associated with that traumatic or stressful event. These studies showed that over time people who had written about their emotions had fewer health problems, a strengthened immune system and a heightened sense of well-being compared with those who had written about a trivial topic. These results have since been repeated several times by many researchers. It doesn't always work, but there is sufficient evidence to show that it is a useful technique that works for many.

We are going to describe a number of different techniques for writing about your traumatic event. What you should do is not necessarily use all these techniques, but have a look through and see which one(s) you would prefer to try. We are separating these into expressive writing and narrative exposure techniques. It may be better to try one of the expressive writing techniques first and see how that works, as narrative exposure involves a far more detailed and complex attempt at writing. The choice also depends on the kind of traumatic event that you have been through. Narrative exposure is particularly useful for those events where there is a perpetrator, where a person has committed some act or crime and was responsible for the traumatic event. It involves the creation of a written testimony that could – in theory, though we are not aware that it has yet happened – be used as a witness statement in court.

Doing expressive writing

What is interesting about the task is that there is usually no audience. The writing is completed and the pages are then thrown away. That makes it unusual among narrative techniques, which usually require an audience, as we have seen. The benefit is that the writer is not compelled to provide any support or backing for what is written; there is no justification for emotions felt or behaviours carried out. Of course, there is still an audience for expressive writing, and that is the person doing the writing. Here we are going to suggest different versions of expressive writing that you can try.

Technique 1: Just writing

The first way of doing expressive writing is the simplest: just write. In order to do this you can use either sheets of paper or a computer – it doesn't matter; just use what is easiest for you. Find yourself a quiet place where you will not be disturbed, think about the traumatic event and then write about it for 20 minutes. Don't stop, don't worry about spelling and grammar, don't worry about good sentence structure. Simply write about the event: write whatever you like. After 20 minutes, stop writing. Then throw it away or delete it. Don't keep it, as either you or someone else may see it and read it. The reason for throwing it away is because you have been free to write whatever you like – you might have written something about someone that you could regret if the work is kept.

The next day do exactly the same thing. Write about the traumatic event for 20 minutes, and then throw away what you have written. Do the same thing on the third day and the fourth day.

In summary, you should write for 20 minutes a day for four consecutive days. Don't worry if you miss a day, just do it the following day. This is the basic expressive writing technique and has been shown to reduce symptoms and make people feel better. There are no constraints on what you write. Just remember to throw away each version once you have completed it.

Technique 2: Guided expressive writing

This is similar to the first technique except that you have some instructions about what to write on each of the four days. You still throw away what you have written. You are going to focus on the traumatic event. If there is more than one traumatic event, write about the one that affects you most. The instructions are:

Day 1

Describe what happened. Include how you and others behaved; describe your emotions and feelings at the time, if relevant; write about how you should have acted. Write in detail about your worst, most emotional memories of the event.

Day 2

Thinking about what you wrote on Day 1, write in detail about the worst traumatic memory: what happened and how you felt at the time. Write about how you feel now. Concentrate on those feelings. Make sure you provide as much detail as possible. How have the feelings changed over time? What effects have the traumatic event had on your life? Include effects on your family, your social life and your working life.

Day 3

Thinking about what you wrote on Day 1 and Day 2, again go through a description of your most traumatic memories and the feelings and emotions associated with those memories. Don't worry if you are repeating what you have already written; that's fine. If you can elaborate on what you have already written and provide more detail, then that's better. You should also again write about the effects the traumatic events have had on your life.

Day 4

Today you should write in a different way. You have written about your traumatic memories and the effects they have had on you. Today you should write about anything positive that has come out of the traumatic event. You may think there is nothing, but consider: perhaps you have a better understanding of the intensity and importance of emotions; perhaps you have found that a particular person has been very supportive and helpful – why was this and how was that person supportive? Perhaps you have different (more complex) views about the meaning of life and death. Today's task can be very difficult, but try to write about the 'good', no matter how obscure it might be.

At the end of each day you should still throw away or delete all the material.

Technique 3: Actively working with the written material

This still involves writing for 20 minutes each day for four days, but this time you are going to develop what you have written. It works best if you are using a computer as you can then edit your document, but you can do it on paper if you prefer. Save each document at the end of each day's session, so by Day 4 you will have three versions.

Day 1

As for Technique 2, describe what happened. Include how you and others behaved, describe your emotions and feelings at the time, if relevant, and write about how you should have acted. Write in detail about your worst, most emotional memories of the event.

Day 2

Spend ten minutes carefully reading through what you wrote on Day 1, thinking about what should be written in more detail, what you have missed out and what you think might be wrong. Then spend 20 minutes editing the document. Don't delete things unless you think they are wrong, but elaborate on what you wrote, add further details, make things more clear. Write about the impact of the traumatic event on your family, friends and work. You should end up with a much longer document.

Day 3

Spend ten minutes reading through the documents produced on Day 1 and Day 2, and again, using the document produced on Day 2, elaborate on what you have written. Add further details; bring in aspects of other traumatic memories if appropriate. Then start thinking about how you have dealt with your memories and feelings, and – importantly – how you could start dealing with these memories and feelings. Continue to write about the impact of the traumatic event on your family, friends and work. Again, your document should be much longer than it was.

Day 4

Spend ten minutes reading the documents produced on the first three days and then, using the document from Day 3, elaborate on what you have written. This time try and focus on the positive outcomes, how your thoughts and feelings have changed and developed in response to the traumatic event. If you don't feel there are many positive aspects, write about how you might begin to deal with the problems and what outcomes you would like.

Once you have completed this exercise, delete all four documents.

Technique 4: Long-term expressive writing

For this technique we would like you to try Technique 3 but do it over a longer time period. This time we would like you to write once a week rather than every day. Keep a copy of the latest document with you – print it out if you are using a computer – and try to think about what you have written during the week; if you think of something you want to add, just note it on the document. Then, at the end of the week, you should have some notes ready for work on your new document. Use the same instructions as for Technique 3.

Murdered daughter

Edward's daughter Amy was murdered while backpacking in Thailand. At first Edward found it extremely difficult to cope. He could only think what a terrible father he had been, and he regretted that he had not spent more time with Amy while she was young because he was running his own business and had to work long hours. He then tried using long-term expressive writing. At first he found it difficult. He initially just sat there chewing his pen, not knowing what to write. His first attempt contained little but his feelings of guilt that he hadn't spent more time with Amy. As the first week progressed, though, he started to wonder why he was focusing on this one thing, rather than on details of the murder or the fact that she was lost for ever. He made some notes. When he looked at them at the start of the next session he found he could write a lot more. He started to write about some of the good times they had spent together, whether it was just a few minutes at the back of his shop chatting about school or the much longer times when they had been together on family holidays or she had spent the summer working for him. Edward realized that his focus was wrong, and over the weeks he found that he was making sense of this feeling of guilt; it ceased to be about what he had supposedly not done in the past and was transformed into a feeling of deep sorrow for what he would not have in the future.

Technique 5: Shared expressive writing

For this technique, the instructions are the same as for Technique 4, again with a week's gap between writing sessions, but involving someone you trust very well, someone with whom you can share the document. In practice, you follow the instructions for Technique 4, but this time, preferably a day or two before your next writing session, share your document with the person and ask for feedback. Do this after each of the first three sessions, and when you are writing try to take the person's perspective into account, even if you do not necessarily agree with it. If he or she says things you don't agree with, try to justify your position by writing about it. You may find the other person is making a valid and useful point.

This is the most difficult of the expressive writing tasks, as it involves another person. It is extremely important that you trust this person, and that he or she treats what you are doing in confidence and promises not to divulge anything to anyone else without your express permission. Remember, the person you choose will always have the details of what you write about, so it is important that you are happy to share this information. In Chapter 3 we discussed the way many traumatized people don't like to share their burden with the people they live with, preferring to keep home as a 'safe' place. Because of this it may be better to choose a good friend for this technique. However, the choice is yours. If your wife or husband is the most appropriate choice, then use her or him. You must also be aware that imparting information about your trauma may affect or hurt the person you are sharing it with. Make sure people know what they are letting themselves in for.

Narrative Exposure Writing (NEW)

Narrative Exposure Therapy (or NET) is a therapeutic technique that was created a few years ago by Frank Neuner and colleagues at the University of Konstanz as a means of treating victims of organized violence. It has since been extended for use with other people. It is a short-term approach based on the principles of cognitive behavioural therapy (CBT) and testimony therapy. Drawing on CBT, it adapts what is known as exposure therapy, where the person is asked to repeatedly talk about the worst traumatic event in detail while re-experiencing the emotions that are associated with the event. During this process, the person experiences a reduction of the PTSD symptoms. This is fairly similar to what should happen during the expressive writing techniques. In addition to this exposure, you are creating a testimony, or witness statement, about the event. During the process of NET, you are writing and rewriting what happened, and once this is completed you sign the final document. If you wish it to be used as a witness statement, your signature will need to be witnessed by another individual to confirm that it is accurate.

Here we are adapting NET as another Guided Narrative Technique, so that instead of being a therapeutic technique with a therapist present to advise and help you throughout the process, you are going through the details by yourself, by following instructions.

We would like to take the opportunity to again warn you about the potential distress that you might feel when going through NEW. If you do feel distress that you find difficult to deal with, you should seek professional help. The process only lasts four days but it can take up several hours a day. It would be preferable to carry out the tasks when you will not be disturbed. If possible, take time off work to do it.

Before you undergo NEW, make sure you understand about the symptoms of traumatic stress, possible accompanying problems, and coping and support. If you have read this book so far you will be aware of these issues and realize that the feelings and thoughts you have are normal after a traumatic event.

Day 1

You should write a very detailed account of your traumatic event, focusing strongly not only on what happened but also on exactly how you felt at the time, and what you were thinking. You are not limited to 20 minutes, as you were with expressive writing; you should spend as long as necessary on this task. When you have drafted your account, go through it very carefully and think what you have missed out. Be very honest. After a traumatic event there are things you cannot remember, so say so. There are other things you do remember, but you might feel that you are too upset to write them down. Try your best to write these things down anyway, and write them in the fullest detail. Here we need you to focus on the worst memories you have, the most intense feelings and your thoughts about what happened. Everything is relevant. If you get upset, try to relax yourself and then get back to writing.

Day 2

Read through your account from the previous day. Don't just skim it: read it very carefully, particularly the parts about the traumatic memories and the feelings. Did you write it accurately? Are there details that you missed out that you now remember? Put these details in. Have you now started to interpret your thoughts and feelings from the time of the traumatic event differently? Add that in at the end. By now you should have produced a document – probably fairly lengthy – that contains very detailed accounts of your traumatic memories, exactly what happened, including causes and consequences, your feelings and thoughts at the time and, in the final part of the document, how you have reinterpreted your thoughts and feelings since that time, right up to the present day. There should also be detailed accounts of how your interactions and relationships with significant others (family, friends, work colleagues) have changed because of the traumatic event. How have they responded? Have there been problems? Detail these.

Day 3

Repeat the process of Day 2. Read the document slowly and carefully, and add in further details as described. This document should now be nearing completion. You may not want to look at it or read it, but do so. If it causes you distress, put it down and relax. Then get back to it.

Day 4

Today you will be producing the final document. Repeat what you have done on previous days, even to correcting spelling and grammar. After all, other people may be reading this document. Once you are happy with the document, print it off and sign it. If you think it could be used as a witness statement, get someone else to witness your signature. The document is then ready for whatever purpose you see fit. If the traumatic event did involve a perpetrator, someone who committed the act, then the statement you have produced could be very useful, certainly as part of the prosecution. Even if the document itself isn't used, it can be the basis for your courtroom account.

May

You will remember May from Chapter 2. She was a survivor of the Szechuan earthquake in 2008. She lost her child and her husband was injured. Initially she didn't have serious psychological problems, but these emerged later, as her husband recovered. Eventually she was unable to work and unable to care for her husband. Her mood was very low and she missed her child enormously. She felt ashamed that she had been unable to keep her alive, that she hadn't been with her at the time. A group of aid workers, which included psychologists, offered treatment using NEW. May agreed to do this as she understood she was ill. She wrote about exactly what happened on the day of the earthquake, and then wrote about her own responses to that. On the second day she looked through the document and made some changes, but really this was just providing more detail. It wasn't until the third day that she included the phrase that it was a 'normal day', which made her think about how she should not have been with her child that day. It was just like any other day until the earthquake struck. While this did not reduce the sense of loss that May felt regarding her child, it did help her deal with the sense of shame she had been feeling about not being there for her.

This case illustrates how using these techniques is not about finding a cure and making you perfectly well. If you have lost a member of your family – perhaps especially if it is a child – there is no way you are going to get over that loss quickly, or ever. What these techniques are trying to do is help you manage the loss more effectively.

Testing yourself

At the end of Chapter 2 we asked you to obtain your scores on the PTSD, anxiety and depression scales, along with the coping scale. Once you have completed one or more of the techniques described here, please do the tests again. If the techniques have helped, your scores should have reduced on the PTSD, anxiety and depression scales (assuming they were high in the first place). Ideally, your coping strategies might have become more adaptive and less maladaptive.

Conclusions

In this chapter we have outlined a number of guided writing techniques that have been shown to reduce symptoms of traumatic stress in people. In one sense these have been somewhat artificial, because most have not had an audience and you have not been writing for someone else. In the next chapter, we look at those methods of writing that do have an audience, when you are writing for and with others.

9

Writing for and with others

While we have touched on using your writing for other people in the previous chapter, this brief chapter will explore other ways in which we use writing to tell other people about ourselves. These include some of the oldest techniques we have, such as letter-writing, and some of the newest, including the internet and email.

Letters

People have for many centuries used letters to tell others about their problems, and this can include problems caused by the stress and trauma in their lives. Though the use of language may be different (the words 'trauma' and 'stress' did not have their current psychological meaning even a hundred years ago), letters down the years contain descriptions of people trying to make sense of the difficult times in their lives.

We still do it today. People 'pour out their troubles' in letters. When writing to someone they describe in great detail things that they would never say face to face. The letter – though since the advent of the internet it is less popular than it used to be – still plays an important role in meaning-making.

The letter is a good way of relieving the symptoms associated with trauma, for those who are able to discuss them, as not only does it take time and effort to write about the traumatic experience (just like the exercises in the previous chapter), but it is written for a familiar audience, probably a friend, who is accustomed to your personal characteristics, and probably also knows about the traumatic event. A letter is – usually – also written in the expectation of a reply: a reply that in this case may provide useful advice and help, and may ask questions that provide you with insight. Once a person answers a letter and includes questions, it is likely that the correspondence will develop further, and there may be several letters from each person. Through this process of explanation and elaboration you can begin to make sense or meaning from what is being described. As the person who is the audience gains a better understanding through asking for clarification or further detail, then you too gain a better understanding.

This happens in a normal conversation, but with two big differences. One we have just mentioned: that many people will write more in a letter than they say face to face; and the second is that you can spend a lot more time composing the written word than the spoken word, and can take more care over the selection of words. Again, this will help in meaning-making.

Email

Email seems to have been with us for ever, but as a mass form of communication it only really got going in the 1990s. To many of us it is trouble; those who sit at desks have new emails arriving constantly, and many of us are not disciplined enough just to answer them at one or two points in the day. It also means that the network of communication has broadened considerably.

On the other hand, email is a very useful form of communication. It is being more widely used for research interviews, because it has the same advantages as the letter described above. The questioner can take time over constructing the questions, and the respondent can take time over constructing replies. This has the effect that the conversation between letter-writers described above can take a matter of hours rather than weeks, even when taking one's time over constructing the emails. This is not necessarily better than letters, as the space of several days between sending a letter and receiving the reply allows one to mull over the problem, to 'sleep on it' as the popular and accurate phrase goes. We do know that many problems get resolved over these periods of time.

Using the internet

There is a vast amount of information available on the internet for helping people who are traumatized. There are websites which provide information about different kinds of traumatic events and the symptoms that result from traumatic experiences. There are websites that discuss the research available about trauma. Then there are many sites where you can interact with other people who share problems. This resource, which like email did not become popular until the 1990s, is now critical in the lives of many of us. The problem with the internet is what it has always been: you do not always know which websites you can trust. The general rule is that if the information is provided by a recognized body, such as the government, the health service, the BBC or a familiar charity, you can probably trust the information, as it will usually have been provided by experts in their field and edited appropriately. That does not mean that other information is not reliable, it just gets more difficult to tell. If, for example, you are finding out about traumatic stress and treatment then you should look at different websites and compare the information.

Discussion forums

One important function of the web for people who are traumatized is the discussion forum. There are many discussion forums about PTSD on the internet. Some of these focus on one specific type of traumatic event; others are more general. They tend to be very informative – though you do need to be careful about how much you can rely on the information as it is not always monitored. They are most helpful because the discussants are people like you; they are people who have similar problems and want to discuss them. These sites can be very effective at providing you with information and also with social support. Another advantage is that they can be anonymous. You do not have to provide your real name and your address. This means you can discuss your problems with other people in a confidential manner – an interesting idea as your comments are available across the internet!

While some forums are not monitored, others are, and these tend to be the best ones, as inappropriate comments can be removed and so can troublemakers. You should explore the different options before deciding which to join. They are also – usually – free of charge.

Social networking

A fairly recent invention of the internet is the social networking site. These are extremely popular, with sites such as Facebook and Twitter having many millions of members. These sites enable people to form groups. These can be any kind of group, and those relating to trauma are popular; as with discussion forums, some of these groups are moderated while others are not. Groups like this function in a similar way to discussion forums, with members providing or asking for information or advice.

Conclusion

This short chapter is unlikely to have told you anything new, but it is here to show that the ordinary everyday ways in which we interact with others via the written word can be very helpful in overcoming trauma. From the simple letter to discussion forums, traumatized people can express their problems and, we hope, receive good information and helpful replies. It is often the people who have had similar experiences who can be most helpful and supportive, because they understand your problems very well – they have the same issues. On the other hand, those who have not had the same experiences can be supportive because they want to understand; by requesting that understanding they are showing you that they care, and they are also giving you the opportunity to write about your problems in great detail, which can be very helpful in increasing your own understanding of those problems. Never dismiss the more common ways of dealing with problems, such as letter-writing; if people have used them for centuries, it is because they work.

10

Drawing on others' trauma narratives

This short chapter illustrates how others have used the written word to express their trauma. It may help those of you who are still having problems expressing yourselves by showing what others have achieved. In this section we focus on the kinds of narratives that people have developed through writing, and talk about some examples.

Much of the world's literature is based on a relatively limited number of universal themes, and these include love, happiness, loss, death and trauma. The best books interweave several of these themes, often developing the sense of tragedy, where something awful happens, and the themes then depend on how the participants resolve the issues that arise from this tragedy. From this – by reading some of the great literature – the reader can develop insight into human nature. Our argument here is that a traumatized person can learn something about his or her own problems, and perhaps ways of dealing with them, by reading relevant literature.

It is not only books: there are plays and films, television series and poetry, all the forms of art that tell us something about human nature. However, while they are very useful in helping us understand the nature of traumatic stress we should bear in mind that they have their limitations. Often they are created as entertainment, and they may oversimplify the ways we respond to traumatic events. Nevertheless they can still provide us with some understanding.

We can go back to Ancient Greece to find examples of traumatic stress: Homer's *Iliad* is a good example of war trauma. Some of the great novelists of the nineteenth century wrote about wartime experiences, such as Tolstoy's account of fighting in the Crimean War in his *Sevastopol Sketches* or the Napoleonic Wars in *War and Peace*, and Zola's account of the Franco-Prussian War in *La Débâcle*.

The First World War generated a lot of literature, including Erich Maria Remarque's *All Quiet on the Western Front* (which we will consider in more detail later), Ernst Jünger's *Storm of Steel*, Ernest Hemingway's *A Farewell to Arms*, Siegfried Sassoon's *Memoirs of an Infantry Officer* and Vera Brittain's *Testament of Youth*. Later fiction about that war, written not by participants but by people born long after the conflict, includes the *Regeneration* trilogy by Pat Barker and Sebastian Faulks' *Birdsong*. The poetry of the war poets, Wilfred Owen, Siegfried Sassoon and others, represents the nature of war as experienced in the trenches.

The Second World War generated even more literature, including a great deal of writing about the Jewish Holocaust, such as Primo Levi describing his experiences in Auschwitz in *If This is a Man* and the months getting home to Italy in *The Truce*, or Anne Frank's diary, kept while in hiding in Amsterdam. Describing the sheer brutality of the war on the Eastern Front, Guy Sajer wrote *The Forgotten Soldier*. The suffering of Berliners, the rape of the women by Russian soldiers, the starvation and killings at the end of the war have all been described in non-fiction by many people, such as Cornelius Ryan (*The Last Battle*), Antony Beevor (*Berlin*) and, from the personal perspective, in the anonymous *A Woman in Berlin*.

Solzhenitsyn wrote about the trauma in Russia during much of the twentieth century, particularly the Soviet years, including his account of the Soviet prison system, *The Gulag Archipelago*; and then there are accounts from wars such as those in Vietnam and Bosnia; for example Zlata Filipović's *Zlata's Diary*, about a girl trying to survive Sarajevo under siege, or *Not My Turn to Die: Memoirs of a broken childhood in Bosnia* by Savo Heleta. In the last decade many accounts of the harrowing fighting in Iraq and Afghanistan have been written, often by participants, whether soldiers or journalists.

There are also many narrative accounts of other traumatic experiences such as child abuse and rape: *I Never Told Anyone: Writings by women survivors of child abuse*, edited by Ellen Bass and Louise Thornton; *Don't Tell Mummy: A true story of the ultimate betrayal*, by Toni Maguire; *After Silence: Rape and my journey back* by Nancy Raine. David Pelzer wrote detailed accounts of child abuse. More recently, Madeleine McCann's mother, Kate, has published an account about the loss of her daughter. Sheila Cassidy wrote an account of her experiences as a prisoner of the Pinochet regime in the early 1970s. Terry Waite, John McCarthy and others wrote books about their experiences as prisoners in Beirut in the 1980s and 1990s. All these accounts show how the ordinary person gets caught up in traumatic and violent experiences.

The list is virtually endless. We list a few at the end of the book, but you can find out about many others via the library or the internet. Here we are going to focus in detail on just one example, to show how it describes traumatic events and people's responses to those events.

All Quiet on the Western Front: Erich Maria Remarque

> A generation of men who, even though they may have escaped its shells, were destroyed by war.

Remarque's book, published in 1929, is one of the best descriptions of the effects of war on men. Although it is a fictional account, it is based on Remarque's experiences on the Western Front in the First World War. The war experiences of the main character, Paul Baumer, and his comrades provide a complex picture of the impact of war on ordinary men. At one level, Remarque recognizes that it is very difficult to describe war events in words: 'Attack, counterattack, charge, repulse – these are words, but what things they signify.' Or, 'the shelling is stronger than everything. It wipes out the sensibilities.' He also recognizes that people who have not been through such events cannot understand them:

> Suddenly my Mother seizes hold of my hand and asks falteringly, 'Was it very bad out there Paul?' Mother, what should I answer to that? You would not understand, you could never realize it. And you never shall realize it.

Remarque describes the differences between the younger soldiers, who signed up straight from school, and the older soldiers, who already had a career and a wife before the war.

> They have a background that is so strong that war cannot obliterate it. We young men of twenty, however, have only our parents, and some, perhaps, a girl – that is not much, for at our

age the influence of parents is at its weakest and girls have not yet a hold over us.

Remarque talks about the way Paul and his comrades use various coping strategies to deal with their experiences.

> Habit is the explanation for why we seem to forget things so quickly . . . They are too grievous for us to be able to reflect on them at once. If we did that, we should have been destroyed long ago. I soon found out this much: terror can be endured so long as a man simply ducks; but it kills if a man thinks about it.

Or again:

> The terror of the front sinks deep down when we turn our backs upon it; we make grim, coarse jests about it, when a man dies, we say he has nipped off his turd, and so we speak of everything; that keeps us from going mad; as long as we take it that way we maintain our own resistance.

Sometimes coping becomes very difficult:

> Rarely does an incident strike out a spark. But then unexpectedly a flame of grievous and terrible yearning flares up. Those are dangerous moments. They show us that the adjustment is only artificial.

The book shows a remarkable understanding of the impact of war and the problems people face during war. Remarque talks about the memories, the difficulties with coping, and the problems associated with families. It is an eloquent expression of using narrative to cope with traumatic memories.

The sequel to *All Quiet on the Western Front*, *The Road Back*, describes how the men adjusted back into civilian life after the war. This book shows the differences between people: how some adjusted quite easily while others had great difficulties dealing with civilian life.

Remarque's personal story is of interest here. We can see how his life was tragic (in the literary sense). For him the precipitant was the war and the suffering in the trenches. Through this came knowledge about people and how they cope with traumatic events. The affirmation stage is Remarque's post-war life, how his books – not just *All Quiet on the Western Front* – described many different facets of people's lives. They are very personal books. It is questionable whether Remarque would have ended up as a great novelist if he had not experienced the trenches of the First World War.

Conclusion

This brief overview of some of the published work of literature and the arts is a very small sample from a huge amount of work that has been written. Much of it is fictional, but there are many thousands of real-life accounts, where traumatized people have written about their experiences, often to help relieve their symptoms. You can gain insight into trauma-related problems by exploring this literature. Some of it will make no sense to you as your responses may be different, but much of it will strike a chord. Seeing that there are some universal psychological responses to traumatic events can give you a sense of shared experience, itself sometimes comforting.

11

Art and narrative

Some people picture the world graphically rather than in words. For them a painting or drawing engenders feelings another person would draw from words. Some struggle to create stories using words, whether they are trying to think about them, discuss them with other people or write them down on paper. That is perfectly normal; we are all very different people. Just because it is difficult to tell a story in words does not mean that one cannot use narrative techniques that are widely used by people – and also by therapists – including drawing, painting, photography, drama and dance. Artworks are essentially narratives, whether a painting about a particular subject, a photograph of a landscape or representational dance. In this chapter, we will outline some of the key areas of non-verbal narrative development to demonstrate how you may use them yourself.

Drawing and painting

Many traumatized people like to express their feelings and thoughts through drawing and painting. We can find many examples of it by both amateur artists and professionals through the years. The medium of drawing or painting does not matter, neither – particularly – does the skill and competence. If you wish to express your trauma via drawing or painting, then do so. Whether or not someone else will see the resultant work is up to you.

One example of a professional painter who used drawings to represent trauma is Goya, who was present in the early nineteenth century when France invaded Spain. The French occupied Madrid and carried out some terrible atrocities on the people. Goya drew some of these images, creating a set of pictures that horrified those who saw them – and that still horrify people today. They depicted scenes of butchery, hanging, shooting and mass rape. While we do not know whether Goya himself was traumatized by what he saw, it is probable that he felt better after telling his story through these simple drawings.

Other examples relating to mental health generally, rather than trauma specifically, include Hogarth's *The Rake's Progress*, William Blake's *Ghost of a Flea* and Charles Doyle's sketches created during a stay in an asylum (he was the father of Arthur Conan Doyle). During the Spanish Civil War Picasso painted *Guernica* as a response to the bombing by the Fascists of the town of that name. He did it to illustrate the trauma of the people, but also to draw the world's attention to what was happening in Spain at that time.

No one is suggesting that you must have the skill of one of these painters in order to express yourself. The important thing is that you draw or paint the thing that is causing you trouble. Whether these are concrete representations of something to do with the traumatic event itself or more abstract representations does not matter. What is important is that it represents something significant to you.

Art therapy

Art therapy has been used for many years to help people who find it difficult to express themselves in words. It has sometimes been used with large groups, such as after the Kosovan refugee crisis in 1998, when art therapists worked with children in the refugee camps, getting them to draw and paint what they had seen. Many drew pictures of the people who had driven them out of their homes; they drew pictures of guns, tanks and aeroplanes. In research looking at the effects of this kind of therapy, it is clear that simply being able to paint or draw personal images of the traumatic event makes people feel better; it reduces the symptoms of PTSD, depression and anxiety. Art therapy is, of course, widely used with adults too.

The sculptor

Karl was born in Poland in 1920. When the Soviets invaded in September 1939 he managed to escape to Hungary. He was then sent back to occupied Poland to buy guns for the resistance. Unfortunately he was caught by the Russians, who tortured him for 11 days before releasing him. On his return to Hungary he was asked to go back to

Poland again. He refused, and the authorities threatened to shoot him for disobeying orders. Luckily, an officer who was a family member got him released. He was then sent to Canada to train as a Spitfire pilot. Unfortunately his ship was sunk by a U-boat in mid-Atlantic and Karl was left on a life-raft for 17 days before being rescued. He survived by holding on to the thought that he had not said goodbye to his mother – nor had he lost his virginity. He fought the rest of the war as a Spitfire pilot, but in the years after the war the life-raft and the experience of torture haunted him and he spent time in an asylum. In the 1950s he became a sculptor. He found that his memories vanished in the chipping away of the stone to create beautiful pieces of art. From beginning sculpting as a hobby he took it on as a profession, and continued to sculpt for the rest of his life.

Photography

Photography is another art form that can help relieve the pressure of traumatic memories. Indeed, in some ways it can be an extension of walking and talking, as described in Chapter 7, as it may involve wandering around the landscape. Don McCullen, who spent many years as a war photographer and who saw and survived some very dangerous situations, ended up taking photographs of landscapes and other peaceful scenes in his retirement. Again, we do not know the degree to which McCullen was traumatized by his war experiences, but it is likely that his later exploration of the beauty of the landscape through photography did help him with his thoughts and feelings regarding war.

You too can use photography to help ease your difficult traumatic memories. The subject of your photographs is up to you, but it may help to take photographs of peaceful and beautiful things such as landscapes, flowers or animals. It is worth getting the best camera you can afford and learning to use it to take good photographs, taking time over preparing each shot and using the capabilities of the camera to its fullest. In recent years digital photography has become readily available at reasonable prices. Furthermore, because you download your photographs on to a computer means they are very much cheaper to process and print. Also, using appropriate software, you can enhance and change the photographs to create the artwork you desire. All of this can be very helpful.

Drama therapy

This is a more difficult area for an individual. Drama usually involves more than one person and is a complex art form that normally involves words and the explicit construction of stories. What we mean here is not the complexities of a Shakespeare play, but the simplicity of constructing a short play illustrating the traumatic event and your thoughts and feelings about it. Drama therapy is usually carried out in groups with one central component being role play, where the individuals involved act out various scenes relating to their trauma. Another route is to use dolls to enact the scenes. The dolls are used to depict the real people involved and you talk through what is happening as you move them.

Dolls and puppets are widely used with traumatized children, who often don't have the words to describe what has happened. By using dolls or puppets they can act out the scene, perhaps also giving the dolls or puppets the words they themselves find difficult to use.

Drama therapy, whether using dolls or people, is appropriate for someone who finds it difficult to tell the story of the trauma; enacting it by movement draws out extra components of the traumatic event, ones that are difficult to express verbally. An alternative to this is dance movement therapy, which is concerned with enacting the traumatic event through dance.

Conclusion

What this short chapter has tried to do is show that narratives are derived not only from words but also from artwork. From cave drawings to *Guernica*, including photography, sculpture, drama and puppetry, narratives of trauma can be created. People have always used artistic representations to better understand themselves and the world around them.

12

Using narratives in groups and communities

While this book is largely about individuals trying to help themselves to get better, there have been numerous instances when we have suggested getting together with another person to discuss the impact of the traumatic event. This arises naturally from the desire we all have to help each other, to help our friends and those in need. It is perfectly natural to want to help someone who has a problem. We have focused mostly on how one other person can help, though we did use the example of internet discussion forums, which can have thousands of members; however, there are many cases of how larger groups can be effective at reducing trauma symptoms, particularly where the group have shared a traumatic experience. Most of these groups are small, anything from three or four people to 15 or 20, but sometimes they may consist of entire communities.

Groups

Most of the groups that form to address trauma symptoms relate to specific forms of therapy. As we shall see in the next chapter, there are many different types of individual therapy. In the same way, there are many types of group therapy. It is not our intention here to discuss therapy in any detail, as it is not the purpose of the book, but it is helpful to think of other narrative routes to recovery.

There are groups that provide each other with support. Apart from the internet groups already discussed, there are groups of like-minded people who get together to discuss their experiences. The most obvious of these are the veterans' associations. While these are not formed specifically to address psychological symptoms, this often does turn into one of their key functions. The first author's research into Second World War veterans has shown that many people use veterans' associations for emotional and practical support. For the latter, it was about the groups providing welfare to men who were now past retirement age and who needed the social services or the health service. The veterans' association was very helpful for this. In terms of emotional support, veterans would often say that meetings would get very emotional when they discussed their war stories. This may be a way of repeating old stories, but it did also demonstrate the importance of comradeship, of having been through something together, of helping and supporting each other. Other disasters such as Hillsborough in Sheffield, the fire at Bradford football ground or the sinking of the *Marchioness* in London, and attacks such as that of Israel on Gaza or Al Qaeda on Washington and New York have led to survivors' groups being formed that provide a very similar service, giving both emotional and practical support.

The difficulty with forming a group relating to traumatic stress generally is that there need to be hard and fast rules, and most successful groups usually have a facilitator, who is usually a therapist. That is not to say a group without a therapist will not work, but the rules must be clear.

From the camps

A group of old men sit together in a circle with a facilitator. The men are all veterans of Second World War Japanese camps. It is a semi-formal group that allows people to join or leave as they wish. Some people stay for a long time; some only turn up for a single session. There are few rules but they are employed strictly, the main one being that only one person tells his story each week. That person is encouraged to speak in detail. The facilitator leads the questions, but everyone is allowed to ask questions. The aim is to enable the person speaking to elaborate his story and to explore his feelings and thoughts. Many people will provide just a factual story at first, one that has been told many times, only discussing thoughts and feelings when directly questioned. The other people cannot talk about their own stories, except as background to a question. Inevitably, many people want to avoid talking about their experiences (even though they have agreed to attend the workshops) and do not turn up for 'their' session, so another rule is that a back-up person must be prepared to speak. As there are relatively few group members, each person gets the chance to tell his story on a regular basis, with the others encouraging elaboration and discussion. New members listen to others' stories first, so they understand the procedure when it is their turn to speak.

This kind of scenario can be very effective. It is very like a group of people sitting around a table discussing their problems. The rules regarding the right of one person to tell his story and for the others to take it in turns during the different weeks mean that everyone gets a chance to speak – which is often not the case in conversations! The structured questions also mean that the story is elaborated; the person is encouraged to talk about his worst memories, with the result that he can 'own' the interpretation that develops. Many people do not like speaking about painful memories, but can be encouraged to do so in a supportive and friendly environment. One last rule is that everything that is said and done in the group is confidential.

Community work

Narratives can also be developed at the community level. Guided Narrative Techniques can apply just as much to communities as to individuals and groups. These techniques are useful if a community has been through a distressing or traumatic event. Examples might include a country torn apart by war, such as Bosnia, Palestine or Iraq, a city subjected to terrorism or a region affected by a natural disaster such as an earthquake, volcanic eruption or tsunami. It is not important that every person was directly involved; within a community, if many people have been involved then they will be the friends and relations of others, and in the end most members of a community will have been affected.

As for smaller groups, it is important that there are rules for the development of the narratives. Each person must have the opportunity both to tell his or her own story and to listen to others. In this way shared experiences and shared thoughts and feelings can be discussed and dealt with. In dealing at the same time with individual and community interpretations a relatively coherent story can develop, one which of course has different voices, as no two people will have identical experiences and responses.

The purpose of community narrative development is threefold. First, it is to help individuals with their own symptoms; second, it is to draw the community together in supportive networks; and third, it is to tell the story of what happened. This final point is important. Having a final objective, perhaps publishing a website or a book about the event, or even organizing an event where the final story is retold, is something positive to aim for from the beginning, and it will encourage those who are reluctant to talk to open up with their thoughts.

The stories can be collected via interview, tape-recorded and transcribed; via public meetings; or via letters and email. The method of collecting the information doesn't matter, but it is important that people get the opportunity to revisit what they have said in the light of their future thinking and in the light of what other people are saying. A project like this will need someone to coordinate it and probably a team of helpers.

Chilean women

When Pinochet came to power in Chile in the coup of 11 September 1973, many people disappeared. No one knew whether they had been killed or imprisoned. The Catholic Church formed group therapy sessions for many of the women family members of the missing, and out of these the women created *arpilleras*, brightly coloured wall hangings depicting intricate scenes and made of rags embroidered on burlap. Many of these *arpilleras* contained photographs, images or names of their missing family members; they were often sent to different communities in an attempt to trace the missing people. This had to be done in secret, as the creation of *arpilleras* was forbidden. Many were sent to other countries to let the world know what Pinochet was doing. The work of these *arpilleristas* – as the women were known – helped the community deal with the difficult situation they found themselves living in. The authors recently visited Chile and saw many examples of these *arpilleras* in a museum in Santiago. They are very beautiful pieces of work.

Conclusion

The purpose of this short chapter is not to encourage you to find groups and work with them, though it might be a good idea to do so if you think it is appropriate. It is simply to show the range of ways narrative can be, and is, used in order to help people with trauma-related problems. As we have already said, narrative techniques are the easiest ones for us to use, as we use them every day. Here we are just providing some guidance about how to use them. Furthermore, this chapter illustrates that with many traumatic experiences people are not alone: they share the experience with others. There can be a sort of collective trauma, a trauma that is best dealt with by talking about it together.

13

The limits of narrative, the need for psychotherapy

This book is about how narrative approaches – storytelling in one form or another – can help people who have been traumatized. Telling stories is the most natural thing that we do as human beings. It is one of the key things that distinguish us from other animals. As we have seen, we use stories in all areas of our lives. They help us to make sense of the world, to give the world meaning. We have seen how there are many different ways of creating and telling stories: that we can talk, read, listen, write, draw, photograph and paint, and that some of us prefer one method and other people prefer other methods. We have seen how people who have been traumatized can use stories to make sense of their world.

However, there are limits to storytelling. Not everyone who is traumatized is able to tell his or her story of the event. For some people, the emotions and feelings are too intense to be able to make sense of what happened, to tell the story. For these people, something more is needed, whether that is drug therapy or psychotherapy. We will describe some of the therapeutic approaches later in the chapter.

What have we achieved?

We have explored a number of different approaches to developing a narrative relating to traumatic memories. These have included everything from just thinking about what the event means, through talking and writing about it, to using art to develop narratives. Many of you will have used these techniques successfully and, we hope, are feeling better because of them. At this level, narrative works. It can help reduce symptoms; it can help you with your thoughts and feelings; it can help you with your relationships with others; but it does not always work and it may not provide everything you need.

What are the limits of narrative?

If you are still having problems, then this is a short but important section. For most of the book we have been arguing the benefits of a narrative approach and trying to show how many of the problems we face as a result of stressful or traumatic experiences can be dealt with by making sense of them, by trying to understand personally what has happened and putting it in the context of other things that have happened.

As we said earlier, if you are traumatized then one of the big problems is that it can fundamentally change your views about the world, about other people and about yourself. Whereas in the past you probably thought fairly positively about all these things, now traumatic events can sometimes make it very difficult to think positively. If you think you behaved badly or inappropriately in the traumatic situation it is not easy to rid yourself of the shame, guilt or anger that you might experience as a result. It is not easy to think that this was an exceptional situation and that you shouldn't blame yourself for what you did or didn't do. Likewise, if the traumatic event had a perpetrator then it is difficult to trust other people in general. It is very difficult to come to the realization that although that person may have done something horrible, most people are on the whole reasonably good.

Another problem with developing a narrative can be the intensity of feelings you experience when you think of the traumatic event. These are often so intense and uncontrollable that it is difficult or impossible to cope, so it is no wonder that many traumatized people will avoid thinking about their traumatic event as much as possible. As we stated earlier, when a traumatic memory is triggered it often triggers the emotional response automatically – that is why the memory is called traumatic. What you are trying to do when making sense of what happened is to separate the emotion from the memory and find ways of coping.

This is both where the narrative is central, in the sense that you must in some way make sense of the traumatic event, and where the narrative is not enough. If you cannot bear to think of the traumatic event then how can you make sense of it? As we have seen in previous chapters, there are many ways of creating narratives, sometimes alone and sometimes with others, but there are occasions when none of these methods will work. That is not because you are weak or incompetent, or because the people you are speaking to, your friends and relations, are not good enough to support you properly: it is because it is simply too difficult to deal with. This is where external professional help can be of great benefit.

Close relationships and jointly constructed narratives

One of the benefits and disadvantages of narratives is that when two people are in a relationship narratives are at least partially jointly constructed. The traumatized person's narrative will affect and be affected by the other person's narrative.

It is often the case that a book such as this one is bought by someone who has a relative or a friend who is traumatized and who appears not to want to get help or to listen to people who are trying to help. This can be a very difficult situation to deal with, and in severe cases relationships are damaged or can break down because of it. This again may be where professional help is necessary.

The problem with relationships is that both people think they know best, they both know what they want and each thinks he or she knows what the other person wants. In good relationships and in normal times this is usually true. We often understand one another very well, and the more we can think about the other's needs – not forgetting our own – the better the relationship.

Unfortunately, a traumatic experience can create severe problems with relationships, particularly if it is something that happened to one person and not the other. The traumatized person is extremely upset, angry, ashamed, guilty, anxious or depressed, and genuinely wants to get better, so both have the same objective. The problem is that the approaches to resolving the problem may not be the same, and this is where conflict arises. If you are the traumatized person you may think your partner doesn't care, or is expecting you to 'get over it' quickly, or that he or she is trying to get you to go to therapy when you are frightened of it. On the other hand, if you are the partner you may believe you are trying to do the best for the traumatized person by getting him or her to talk. Talking is good for you – we have said this several times in this book – but talking is not *always* good for someone, and people may be very careful about whom they choose to talk to. We have given good reasons why traumatized people might not want to talk to their direct family, because they want to keep the family as a safe environment. No one should be forced to talk about traumatic memories; you have to want to talk. If your partner is asking you to go to therapy and you do not want to talk, then it may be the wrong time for therapy.

These are simple examples, but this is how relationships can go wrong. Both partners think they are doing the right thing, and each wants to help the other, but when communication breaks down like this it can be tremendously difficult. The partner may normally be a very patient person, but there is a limit to what anyone can put up with. The partner may be providing what he or she hopes is good support, but if it is not perceived as such by the traumatized person then it is not good support.

What we have is the traumatic event intruding into people's closest relationships. If the two of you cannot sort this out it is very helpful to get the perspective of someone from outside – often a friend, but friends are not necessarily the right choice as they have complex relationships with you. It may be best to go to relationship counselling, where a neutral professional counsellor will be in a better position to work out what is going on and offer some helpful advice on what to do about the problems.

Where do you go from here?

If, after working through the previous chapters, you are still having significant and serious problems relating to your traumatic memories then you may find counselling or psychotherapy helpful. The best way to do this is often through your GP, who can advise and make recommendations for help from different types of counsellors and psychotherapists (including psychiatrists if there is a need for drug treatment, perhaps for anxiety), though you can of course bypass your GP and seek help privately from a therapist. You can find many different kinds of therapist via the internet, your local library or the Yellow Pages. If you take this route you are advised to find someone who is properly qualified to undertake the therapy or counselling. This can usually be ascertained by checking the appropriate professional body, such as the British Psychological Society or the British Association for Counselling and Psychotherapy. There is a list of addresses at the end of the book.

What are the options?

Counselling and psychotherapy

There are many forms of counselling and therapy. It is difficult to recommend any particular form as people are very different, have different needs and so benefit from different kinds of professional help. We have looked at some of these therapies in earlier chapters, particularly forms of narrative therapy, and how they can help people. In the end all talking therapies are about narrative, about making sense of the traumatic event. Types of therapy include cognitive behavioural therapy (CBT), eye movement desensitization and reprocessing (EMDR), psychoanalytic psychotherapy, humanistic therapy and, of course, the narrative therapies. Reviews of the literature have shown that CBT, EMDR and Narrative Exposure Therapy are all effective, though bear in mind that none work with everyone, and that if a therapy is going to work you must want to be treated. Therapy can be very painful, as it involves dealing with the traumatized memories and the associated emotions.

The idea that people are different and so need different approaches is important. People have in the past assumed that a particular therapy will work for everyone. We know that is not the case, but the health authorities in the United Kingdom do make recommendations. The therapies that are recommended include CBT and EMDR, which are described on pp. 94–5. While it is the case that these are good therapies, we must repeat they do not work for everyone. For instance, there is a lot of evidence that CBT works very well for people who go through the full course of treatment, but the treatment can be very brutal and difficult and many people just cannot complete it. Other therapies, which may not have such good scientific evidence for their effectiveness, can nevertheless be effective for the right person. While you are reading through the therapies described in the rest of this chapter (and it is not a comprehensive account – there are so many therapies available it would take another book to describe them), try to think what kind of approach appeals to you; then, when you go to the GP or when you decide to go privately to a therapist or counsellor, you will have some understanding of the kind of help you would like to receive.

Assessment

Before any therapy takes place, you should have a detailed assessment. This is particularly necessary for traumatic stress as the disorder can be so complex, and the therapist must make sure that he or she is treating the right symptoms. The elements of the assessment may include:

- working out the nature of the traumatic stressor (what actually happened);
- establishing your role in the event;
- your thoughts and feelings about actions taken and not taken during the event;
- the effect of the trauma on your life;
- how you feel about yourself and others;
- whether you have been exposed to prior traumatic events;
- the ways you normally cope with stressful times in your life;
- whether you are able to concentrate and think normally when doing other things, e.g. working;
- your personal strengths and weaknesses;
- any record of previous mental health problems;
- your relevant medical, social, family and occupational history (e.g. relationship issues, unemployment, severe illness);
- your cultural and religious beliefs.

This assessment may take a couple of hours or more, but it is critical that it is done in such detail.

Once the assessment has been carried out a treatment plan can be devised. The treatment plan is highly individualistic: it depends on the needs of the person concerned. It is likely that different types of therapy will be used at different stages of the treatment process, as there are likely to be several different problems to deal with, such as high levels of anxiety, problems with the traumatic memory, and often the kinds of distorted beliefs traumatized people have (e.g. thinking that the world is an unsafe place).

Now let's briefly explore some of the more common therapies available.

Cognitive behavioural therapy (CBT)

CBT is widely used for the treatment of trauma, and it works best as trauma-focused CBT, where the therapeutic techniques are linked to the trauma itself rather than being general techniques. There are several elements to CBT, with the focus being – as it says in the name – cognitive and behavioural techniques. The behavioural techniques are used to deal with the anxiety and fear associated with the traumatic memory. Typically this will involve the person being exposed to the traumatic memory, whether by being taken to the site where the event took place or – more likely – being asked to recall it in detail. Before this exposure the therapist will have taught the person to relax, so that during the exposure these relaxation techniques can be used. Repeated exposure will then – theoretically – lead to a reduction in the association between the fear and anxiety and the memory, enabling the person to cope with any reminders of the memory.

The cognitive element of treatment can be about teaching the person to identify trauma-related unhelpful beliefs and to challenge and modify them. For instance, someone who has been raped may not trust any man – including her husband. This is a very unhelpful belief as it is likely to be damaging to relationships and will also lead to the person being frightened every time she meets a man. Challenging this belief may involve asking her to think about why she holds the belief, and then to think of the evidence that she has for the belief. This should lead to an understanding that men can generally be trusted, and that to think of them all as potential rapists is not helpful for her living her own life.

Eye movement desensitization and reprocessing (EMDR)

EMDR was introduced in the 1980s and was at first distrusted by many therapists, but it quickly became established as a mainstream therapy and there is a lot of evidence that it works. EMDR involves a number of strategies; some are similar to CBT, but one key difference is that you are asked to think about your traumatic event while watching a finger (or pencil, or line on a computer screen, etc.) moving rapidly back and forth in front of your eyes. The object acts as a distractor, enabling you to learn to think about your traumatic experience without experiencing the fear and anxiety that you have normally felt. The exact mechanism of EMDR is not known.

Humanist therapy

Humanist therapies ultimately derive from the philosophies of existentialism and phenomenology and focus on a holistic approach to the person, specifically dealing with how we construct personal meaning in life and exploring our values. It is about taking personal responsibility. One of the pioneers of this area was Carl Rogers, with his person-centred approach to therapy. According to Rogers, the role of the therapist is not to dictate how someone should behave but to listen to people and let them derive their own sense of meaning from their situation. Rogers strongly believed in the person as being at the centre of his or her experience, and that life was continually developing and changing according to the individual's interaction with the world. This makes everyone unique. According to Rogers, a therapist should practise what he called 'unconditional positive regard', i.e. not making any negative judgements about the person. Rogers talked about the fully functioning person, who would have a growing openness to experience and a recognition of the importance of living in the moment, accepting and adapting the personality to experience.

Narrative therapy

We have already looked at how narrative approaches to therapy can help you deal with traumatic memories. Narrative therapy was developed through the 1970s and 1980s, and in some ways it is similar to humanistic therapy, as the therapist is trying to help the patient discover and develop rich narratives that help explain that person's problems. Fundamentally, if you are traumatized you have, according to narrative therapists, a series of 'thin' narratives that explain your predicament. These thin narratives should be replaced by 'thick' narratives that provide a more effective explanation for your experiences. The motto for narrative therapy is 'The person is not the problem, the problem is the problem', which again, like humanistic therapy, shows that it is not the person who is 'bad' or 'wrong'; it is the interpretation of his or her experience. Narrative therapy is about discovering a better interpretation of experience.

Art therapy

We introduced this in Chapter 11. Many people use art as a means of dealing with their traumatic experiences. Art therapy is also a formal therapy, widely used with people who prefer to express themselves artistically rather than using words. As we have seen, art therapy uses a wide variety of techniques: drawing, painting and photography, along with sculpture, puppetry or drama. The art therapist is trained to have a broad understanding of the creative process and how it interacts with psychology. Art can be seen as an external impression of internal psychological processes. Art therapy is particularly effective for people who are not very good at verbal expression. Drama therapy is a form of art therapy that focuses specifically on drama, puppetry and other improvised storytelling techniques. Art and drama therapy are widely used with children, as children may find it easier to express themselves through play rather than words.

Psychoanalysis

There are many types of psychoanalysis, originally derived from the work of Sigmund Freud but developed in many different ways. The therapeutic sessions are designed so that unconscious patterns can be brought into conscious awareness and changed. Freudian techniques such as free association and dream analysis are used. The analyst interprets the patient's responses to provide insight and to help resolve problems. According to Freud, unacceptable thoughts are repressed in childhood and then emerge later as psychological conflict, anxiety or depression; he believed that these repressed thoughts need to be brought into consciousness and reinterpreted so that the problems are removed. Psychoanalysis has been heavily criticized over the years, both for taking a very long time and because there is little evidence for its effectiveness. Nevertheless, many people undergo analysis and believe they benefit from it.

Relationship counselling

As we have seen, traumatic events can damage relationships. Sometimes the most appropriate help might be for not only the traumatized person but also his or her partner to attend. Relationship counselling can help both parties understand the trauma, and also understand the needs of each other. The purpose is to limit the damage the traumatic event has caused to the relationship, enabling social support processes to work more effectively.

General counselling

Counselling is widely available. GPs' surgeries often offer counselling for people in distress. Just as with the types of psychotherapy discussed above, there are many different types of counsellors. Counsellors listen; they tend not to use the wide variety of techniques described above. They generally leave it to you to do the talking and to work through the problem, to develop the meaning or narrative.

Psychiatry

Usually, traumatized people are treated with some form of psycho-therapy as described, but sometimes people are so badly traumatized that they need some extra help. This is the case where someone is so anxious, so worried, that he or she can't deal with the process of psychotherapy. In these cases, anxiolytic drugs are used to reduce the anxiety so that psychotherapy can be used.

Because the symptoms of trauma are so complex, there is no single drug that can be used to treat them all. It may be that drugs are used not to treat PTSD but to treat associated disorders such as generalized anxiety or depression. There are drugs that will help with these things, and drugs that will help the person bring out a repressed traumatic memory.

Some of the more widely used drugs include:

- Selective serotonin uptake inhibitors (SSRIs). There is evidence that this class of drugs is the most effective for reducing PTSD symptoms. SSRIs are generally used in the treatment of depression.
- Monoamineoxidase inhibitors (MAOs). These can improve sleep, reduce the startle response and decrease the level of intrusive thoughts.
- Adrenergic blocking agents such as propranolol and clonidine. These decrease physiological arousal, reduce the startle response, improve sleep, reduce the level of nightmares and reduce the level of intrusive thoughts.
- Lithium carbonate. This is not so widely used but can reduce anger and anxiety.
- Minor tranquillizers such as diazepam and the benzodiazepines. These can control the explosive effects of the traumatic memory, but there is a high risk of dependence.
- D-cycloserine (DCS). This is used to treat tuberculosis, but it also prevents feelings of fearfulness and so helps people to deal with their painful memories constructively, and to unlearn the fear response.
- Yohimbine. This is used to facilitate the recall of traumatic mem-ories, although it can have severe side effects such as intense anxiety.

Psychologists and counsellors cannot prescribe drugs. These can only be prescribed by a medical practitioner such as your GP or a psychiatrist. In an ideal world there will be coordination between the various professionals who will be dealing with a case of traumatic stress: the GP will refer you to the clinical psychologist or other psychotherapist or counsellor, and if there is a need for drug treatment, that will be discussed in conjunction with a psychiatrist. Once the drug treatment is in place, the psychotherapy can then be conducted. In the real world, this coordination may not take place, but you should still discuss your needs with the GP, who is in a position to refer you appropriately.

Conclusions

If, for whatever reason, you are unable to help yourself, there are plenty of options for professional help. Psychiatrists, clinical psychologists, counsellors and other therapists are all available to help. There are many different types of therapy that you can have; there is good evidence that some of them work, but bear in mind that they work for some people and not others. What suits one person may not suit another. Similarly, just because there is limited good evidence that psychoanalysis is effective does not mean it won't be effective for you. In conjunction with obtaining advice from your GP and others you need to decide what approach might suit you best.

14

Conclusions

After a traumatic event, there are several types of response from people. There are some people who walk away and are fine. Others walk away and experience a few problems for a few days or weeks and then recover. Yet others walk away and seem to be all right, but then, perhaps months or even years later, the symptoms start. The final group – fortunately a minority of people – are traumatized.

Most people recover quite well and quite quickly. To experience bad dreams, to cry, to experience fear and other emotions, is perfectly normal after such an event. The problems arise when these do not go away. That is when you may need some help, whether that comes through reading books like this, seeing a professional therapist or talking to a family member or friend.

The intention of this book is not to find some magical cure-all for traumatic stress but to introduce you to ways of helping yourself when you have a problem and finding help where needed. The focus has been on narrative – stories – because over the years it has been shown consistently that helping people to make sense of their experiences is often the first stage to recovery. We do not claim that using these approaches is guaranteed to work – and they won't work unless you make an effort. Indeed, if you have severe problems it is likely that you will need to seek professional help (there are addresses at the end of the book which will help you find appropriate help). People who are severely traumatized are unlikely to be able to make sense of their situation if they are experiencing high levels of distress, having problems with drink and drugs, or having problems with relationships.

In recent years, there has been a growing recognition that for some people trauma symptoms start gradually months or years after the event. For a time many people will be experiencing some problems but do not necessarily have a diagnosis of PTSD. At this stage narrative methods are ideal. It is now, when you are not overwhelmed by symptoms of anxiety, that you can use these methods to help reduce the symptoms that exist and to stop them from getting worse. At the other end of the scale, if your symptoms are so severe that you cannot talk about the event, then you may need therapy for the anxiety before attempting to try the narrative methods. Whatever your situation, if you do not feel ready to try and put your experiences into words (or art) then you are not ready for this book. It takes a strong will to use these exercises to their best advantage, and many of us find it very difficult. Just remember, there is a lot of help available if you need it, from family and friends to a variety of professional therapists and counsellors.

Traumatic stress is a complex set of disorders, not a single disorder called PTSD. The way we respond depends on what happened, on our responses at the time and afterwards, on our personalities and coping styles, and on the types of social support we get from our friends and relatives. There is no pill that will cure everything, and for some traumatic events, such as the death of a child, there will be no full recovery. Nevertheless, a set of simple pointers can make a big difference. We have focused on narrative because, as we have said on several occasions, it is a natural skill, something we do a lot of the time, so it is not something new to learn. The purpose of the Guided Narrative Techniques has been to illustrate how you can adapt and improve your own narrating skills in relation to traumatic stress.

What has this book shown?

We started off by discussing the nature of traumatic events, and then moving on to the individual characteristics that may influence whether or not you are traumatized, specifically personality, coping styles and the support you receive from family and friends. We then showed what we mean by narrative and how we use it in everyday life. After the warning about the dangers inherent in thinking, writing or talking about your traumatic memories we introduced a range of Guided Narrative Techniques. We did this to introduce you to a range of techniques that can usefully help improve your trauma narratives. Recognizing that everyone is different, we provided a range of techniques that included not only thinking, writing and talking, but also art and drama, and the use of GNTs in groups. Finally, for some people these techniques may not have worked, so we briefly discussed the limitations of narrative and provided some details of potential therapies. It is hoped that this will have given you a good understanding of the basics of narrative and how it is used both in everyday life and when you are traumatized.

Finally, remember that no technique will return you to the way you were before the traumatic event. Your life narrative has been disrupted by the event. You now need to find the best way of reconstructing this narrative, incorporating what you have experienced and what you have learned from those experiences.

Appendix A: Measures

The final part of the book contains some information that we hope you will find useful. This appendix provides a series of self-report measures, so that you can explore your own symptoms relating to a number of trauma-related problems, along with a measure of how you cope.

Self-report measures

The following measures are designed to give you some idea of the extent of your problems, and how your symptoms change over time.

It is important to note that these measures are not a substitute for a full assessment for any of the disorders. They provide a guide to whether you may have a disorder. The scores do not infer a medical diagnosis of the disorder, no matter how high the score. Only a fully qualified practitioner (e.g. clinical psychologist or psychiatrist) can provide such a diagnosis.

The measures for PTSD, depression, generalized anxiety and substance abuse relate to the diagnostic criteria for those disorders. They are not reliable and valid standardized scales. If you need further information about whether or not you may have these disorders, please see your medical practitioner.

These scales are included for your information, and also so that you can see whether your scores change over time and when you have completed some of the GNTs. Please answer the measures honestly.

Measure 1: Post-traumatic stress disorder

Criterion A: The stressor

1 Have you experienced, witnessed or been confronted   YES/NO
   with an event or events that involve actual or
   threatened death or serious injury, or a threat to
   the physical integrity of yourself or others?

2 Did your response involve intense fear, helplessness   YES/NO
   or horror? Note: in children, it may be expressed
   instead by disorganized or agitated behaviour.

Criterion B: Intrusive recollection

Do you experience:

3 Recurrent and intrusive distressing recollections of   YES/NO
   the event, including images, thoughts or
   perceptions? Note: in young children, repetitive
   play may occur in which themes or aspects of the
   trauma are expressed.
4 Recurrent distressing dreams of the event? Note: YES/NO
   in children, there may be frightening dreams
   without recognizable content.
5 Acting or feeling as if the traumatic event were   YES/NO
   recurring (includes a sense of reliving the
   experience, illusions, hallucinations and
   dissociative flashback episodes, including those
   that occur upon awakening or when intoxicated)?
   Note: in children, trauma-specific re-enactment
   may occur.
6 Intense psychological distress at exposure to   YES/NO
   internal or external cues that symbolize or resemble
   an aspect of the traumatic event?
7 Physiological reactions when exposed to internal   YES/NO
   or external cues that remind you of an aspect of
   the traumatic event?

Criterion C: Avoidant/numbing

Do you experience the following?

8 Efforts to avoid thoughts, feelings, or conversations   YES/NO
   associated with the trauma
9 Efforts to avoid activities, places or people that   YES/NO
   arouse recollections of the trauma
10 Inability to recall an important aspect of the trauma   YES/NO
11 Markedly diminished interest or participation in   YES/NO
   significant activities

12 Feeling of detachment or estrangement from others YES/NO
13 Restricted range of affect (e.g. unable to have loving YES/NO
feelings)
14 Sense of foreshortened future (e.g. 'I do not expect YES/NO
to have a career, marriage, children, a normal life
span')

Criterion D: Hyper-arousal
Do you experience the following?

15 Difficulty falling or staying asleep YES/NO
16 Irritability or outbursts of anger YES/NO
17 Difficulty concentrating YES/NO
18 Hyper-vigilance YES/NO
19 Exaggerated startle response YES/NO

Criterion E: Duration
20 Have you experienced the symptoms described YES/NO
in Criteria B, C and D for more than one month?

Criterion F: Functional significance
21 Have your symptoms caused significant distress or YES/NO
impairment to your social, occupational or other
important areas of functioning?

Specify whether:
Acute: if duration of symptoms is less than three months

Chronic: if duration of symptoms is three months or more

With or without delayed onset: onset of symptoms at least six
months after the stressor.

Scoring
Criterion A   you must have answered YES to both questions 1
and 2.
Criterion B   you must have answered YES to at least one from
questions 3–7.
Criterion C   you must have answered YES to at least three from
questions 8–14.

Criterion D	you must have answered YES to at least two from questions 15–19.
Criterion E	you must have answered YES to question 20.
Criterion F	you must have answered YES to question 21.

If you have answered yes as indicated above for Criteria A–F then you may have PTSD. You can also see whether it is acute, chronic or delayed onset.

As already indicated, self-report is only an indicator, not a diagnosis. An accurate diagnosis can be obtained from a psychologist or psychotherapist.

Measure 2: Depression

There are many types of depression, and varying degrees of severity. The diagnostic indicator provided below is for your information and does not indicate with certainty whether you have clinical depression, nor does it cover the range of different types of depression.

Please indicate which of the following you have experienced during the same two-week period, and which represent a change from previous functioning (do not count those relating to another physical health problem). This can be scored either by the person or by someone who has observed the person regularly.

Criterion A

1 Depressed mood most of the day, nearly every day   YES/NO
   (e.g. feeling sad or tearful) (note: in children and
   adolescents, can be irritable mood)
2 Markedly diminished interest or pleasure in all, or   YES/NO
   almost all, activities most of the day, nearly every
   day
3 Significant weight loss when not dieting, or weight   YES/NO
   gain (e.g. a change of more than 5 per cent of
   body weight in a month), or decrease or increase
   in appetite nearly every day (note: in children,
   consider failure to make expected weight gains)
4 Sleeping too little or too much nearly every day   YES/NO
5 Psychomotor agitation (restlessness) or retardation   YES/NO

(slowing down of physical and mental faculties)
nearly every day

6	Fatigue or loss of energy nearly every day	YES/NO
7	Feelings of worthlessness or excessive or inappropriate guilt (which may be delusional) nearly every day (not merely self-reproach or guilt about being sick)	YES/NO
8	Diminished ability to think or concentrate, or indecisiveness, nearly every day	YES/NO
9	Recurrent thoughts of death (not just fear of dying), recurrent suicidal ideation without a specific plan, or a suicide attempt or a specific plan for committing suicide	YES/NO

Criterion B

The symptoms cause clinically significant distress or   YES/NO
impairment in social, occupational or other
important areas of functioning

Criterion C

The symptoms are not due to the direct   YES/NO
physiological effects of a substance (e.g. a drug of
abuse, a medication) or a general medical condition
(e.g. hypothyroidism)

Interpretation

In order to be classified as having depression, you should have
answered YES to five or more of the questions in Criterion A,
including either question 1 (depressed mood) or question 2 (loss of
interest or pleasure), and YES to Criteria B and C.

Measure 3: Anxiety

Again, the diagnostic indicator provided below is for your information and does not indicate with any certainty whether you have
anxiety, nor does it cover the range of different types of anxiety.

Please indicate which of the following you have experienced
during the same two-week period and which represent a change

from previous functioning (do not count those relating to another physical health problem). This can be scored either by the person or by someone who has observed the person regularly.

1 Do you have excessive anxiety about a number of events or activities, occurring more days than not, for at least six months?   YES/NO
2 Do you find it difficult to control that worry?   YES/NO
3 Is the anxiety and worry associated with the following:
   (a) restlessness or feeling keyed up or on edge   YES/NO
   (b) being easily fatigued   YES/NO
   (c) difficulty concentrating or mind going blank   YES/NO
   (d) irritability   YES/NO
   (e) muscle tension   YES/NO
   (f) sleep disturbance   YES/NO
4 Is the anxiety about a specific problem, for   YES/NO
   instance social phobia, gaining weight or a serious illness?
5 Does the anxiety cause significant distress or   YES/NO
   impairment in your social or work life?
6 Does the anxiety occur specifically during events   YES/NO
   such as alcohol use or as part of a medical condition?

Interpretation

In order to be classified as having generalized anxiety disorder, you should have answered YES to questions 1 and 2, YES to at least three of the options in question 3, NO to question 4, YES to question 5 and NO to question 6, though again bear in mind this is not a medical diagnosis.

Measure 4: Substance abuse

Have the following occurred over the last 12 months?

1 Recurrent substance use resulting in a failure to   YES/NO
   fulfil your major work or social obligations
   (e.g. absence from work/school)

2   Recurrent substance use in situations that are   YES/NO
    dangerous (e.g. driving a car)
3   Recurrent substance use legal problems (e.g. being   YES/NO
    arrested or charged with offences)
4   Continued substance use despite having social   YES/NO
    or personal problems relating to the substance use

Interpretation

In order to be classified as having substance abuse (not a medical diagnosis) you need to answer YES to all four questions.

Measure 5: Coping

This scale (© Carver, 1997) deals with the ways you cope with the stress in your life. There are many ways to try to deal with problems. Each item says something about a particular way of coping. The scale looks at the extent to which you've been doing each item, how much or how frequently. Don't answer on the basis of whether it seems to work or not – just whether or not you do it. Use these response choices and try to rate each item separately in your mind from the others. Make your answers as true as you can.

1 = I haven't been doing this at all.
2 = I've been doing this a little bit.
3 = I've been doing this a medium amount.
4 = I've been doing this a lot.

1   I've been turning to work or other activities to take my mind off things.
2   I've been concentrating my efforts on doing something about the situation I'm in.
3   I've been saying to myself, 'This isn't real.'
4   I've been using alcohol or other drugs to make myself feel better.
5   I've been getting emotional support from others.
6   I've been giving up trying to deal with it.
7   I've been taking action to try to make the situation better.
8   I've been refusing to believe that it has happened.
9   I've been saying things to let my unpleasant feelings escape.
10 I've been getting help and advice from other people.

11 I've been using alcohol or other drugs to help me get through it.

12 I've been trying to see it in a different light, to make it seem more positive.

13 I've been criticizing myself.

14 I've been trying to come up with a strategy about what to do.

15 I've been getting comfort and understanding from someone.

16 I've been giving up the attempt to cope.

17 I've been looking for something good in what is happening.

18 I've been making jokes about it.

19 I've been doing something to think about it less, such as going to movies, watching TV, reading, daydreaming, sleeping or shopping.

20 I've been accepting the reality of the fact that it has happened.

21 I've been expressing my negative feelings.

22 I've been trying to find comfort in my religion or spiritual beliefs.

23 I've been trying to get advice or help from other people about what to do.

24 I've been learning to live with it.

25 I've been thinking hard about what steps to take.

26 I've been blaming myself for things that happened.

27 I've been praying or meditating.

28 I've been making fun of the situation.

The scale measures your score on a number of coping strategies. There is no overall score, but you might find it helpful to see which coping strategies you tend to use and which you don't. There are two items per coping strategy, as shown below. Add up the scores per strategy, as indicated. A high score is 6–8, a low score is 2–4. There is no 'normal' pattern of responding. We all use different methods of coping – some work better for some of us, others work better for other people.

Self-distraction	items 1 and 19
Active coping	items 2 and 7
Denial	items 3 and 8
Substance use	items 4 and 11
Use of emotional support	items 5 and 15

Use of instrumental support   items 10 and 23
Behavioural disengagement   items 6 and 16
Venting   items 9 and 21
Positive reframing   items 12 and 17
Planning   items 14 and 25
Humour   items 18 and 28
Acceptance   items 20 and 24
Religion   items 22 and 27
Self-blame   items 13 and 26

Measure 6: Post-traumatic growth

The PWB–PTCQ (© Stephen Joseph and Steve Regel, 2009) consists of 18 items. You should rate how much you perceive yourself to have changed on each item as a result of your traumatic experience on a five-point scale:

5 = Much more so now
4 = A bit more so now
3 = I feel the same about this as before
2 = A bit less so now
1 = Much less so now

1 I like myself.
2 I have confidence in my opinions.
3 I have a sense of purpose in life.
4 I have strong and close relationships in my life.
5 I feel I am in control of my life.
6 I am open to new experiences that challenge me.
7 I accept who I am, with both my strengths and limitations.
8 I don't worry what other people think of me.
9 My life has meaning.
10 I am a compassionate and giving person.
11 I handle my responsibilities in life well.
12 I am always seeking to learn about myself.
13 I respect myself.
14 I know what is important to me and will stand my ground, even if others disagree.
15 I feel that my life is worthwhile and that I play a valuable role in things.

16 I am grateful to have people in my life who care for me.
17 I am able to cope with what life throws at me.
18 I am hopeful about my future and look forward to new possibilities.

Three items reflect each of the domains of self-acceptance (1, 7 and 13), autonomy (2, 8 and 14), purpose in life (3, 9 and 15), relationships (4, 10 and 16), sense of mastery (5, 11 and 17) and personal growth (6, 12 and 18). When you total these you have a score of between 3 and 15 for each domain, and a possible range of 18 to 90, with higher scores indicating greater positive change.

Appendix B: Table of options

The following is a quick indicator of the types of Guided Narrative Techniques and whether they use thinking, writing, talking or non-verbal activities. It may help when you are deciding which to use. As you can see, they all involve thinking!

	Thinking	Writing	Talking	Non-verbal
Walking	YES		YES	YES
Guided writing	YES	YES		
Writing for others	YES	YES		
Using published work	YES			
Art and drama groups and communities	YES	YES	YES	YES

Useful addresses

The following lists are not comprehensive. There are many thousands of books, films, plays and poems that have dealt with traumatic stress. Furthermore, there are hundreds of books, thousands of journal articles and many websites dedicated to increasing our understanding of traumatic stress. What follows is a brief compilation of some of those that we think are particularly useful. Most of the websites given provide not only information themselves about traumatic stress but also links to other useful sites.

Therapy information

Your first port of call for therapy is usually your GP, but it can help to learn something about the different therapies that are available.

British Association for Behavioural and Cognitive Psychotherapies
Imperial House
Hornby Street
Bury
Lancs BL9 5BN
Tel.: 0161 705 4304
Website: www.babcp.com
The main organization dealing with CBT practitioners, and providing accreditation.

British Association of Counselling and Psychotherapy
BACP House
15 St John's Business Park
Lutterworth
Leics LE17 4HB
Tel.: 01455 883300
Website: www.bacp.co.uk
Represents many counsellors and psychotherapists across the UK.

British Psychological Society
St Andrew's House
48 Princess Road East
Leicester LE1 7DR
Tel.: 0116 254 9568
Website: www.bps.org.uk
The key organization for psychologists in the UK. Here you will find details of clinical psychologists and others interested in traumatic stress.

EMDR Association United Kingdom and Ireland
PO Box 3356
Swindon SN2 9EE
Website: www.emdrassociation.org.uk
Here you can find details about EMDR (Eye Movement Desensitization and Reprocessing) therapy and EMDR practitioners.

The Institute of Psychoanalysis
Byron House
112A Shirland Road
London W9 2EQ
Tel.: 020 7563 5000
Website: www.psychoanalysis.org.uk
The home of the British Psychoanalytic Society: for those interested in psychoanalytic treatment.

General websites

Alcohol issues
www.alcoholissues.co.uk
Supplies information about alcohol and alcohol misuse; publishes a newsletter.

Association for Counselling and Psychotherapy Online
www.acto-uk.org
Gives details of practitioners who provide online therapy.

David Baldwin's Trauma Pages
www.trauma-pages.com
Provides general information about traumatic stress.

European Society for Traumatic Stress Studies
www.estss.org
Brings together practitioners and researchers in the area of traumatic stress.

International Society for Traumatic Stress Studies
www.istss.org
An international organization for professionals dealing with traumatic stress.

United States Department of Veterans' Affairs
www.ncptsd.va.gov
Provides a site with advice about PTSD: www.ncptsd.va.gov/ncmain/index/jsp. In addition, the Department publishes a PILOTS database which lists the scientific publications relating to PTSD: www.ncptsd.va.gov/ncmain/publications/pilots

World Health Organization
www.who.int/en/
Gives useful information about general health, including PTSD.

Veterans' organizations

Combat Stress
Tyrwhitt House
Oaklawn Road
Leatherhead
Surrey KT22 0BX
Tel.: 01372 587000 (General enquiries); 0800 138 1369 (24-hour helpline)
Website: www.combatstress.org.uk
Assists veterans from the armed forces and their relatives. Clinical short-term treatment is provided at 3 residential centres in Ayrshire, Shropshire and Surrey. There is also a community outreach service.

Help for Heroes
Unit 6, Aspire Business Centre
Ordnance Road
Tidworth
Hants SP9 7QD
Tel.: 0845 673 1760
Website: www.helpforheroes.org.uk
A charity set up in 2007 to help services personnel wounded in Britain's current conflicts.

Royal British Legion
199 Borough High Street
London SE1 1AA
Tel.: 08457 725725 (general enquiries)
Website: www.britishlegion.org.uk
Committed to the welfare and interests of ex-armed services personnel. There are regional offices around the country.

Soldiers, Sailors, Airmen and Families Association (SSFA Forces Help)
19 Queen Elizabeth Street
London SE1 2LP
Tel.: 0845 1300 975 (general)
Forcesline: 0800 731 4880 (freephone available 10.30 a.m. till 10.30 p.m. (UK local time): for any rank to talk things through in confidence on any issue.
Website: www.ssafa.org.uk
SSAFA Forces Help provides assistance for anyone serving in the armed forces or for anyone who has ever served. The Forcesline is also available for armed forces personnel serving in various places around the world.

Other organizations

Addaction
67–69 Cowcross Street
London EC1M 6PU
Tel.: 020 7251 5860
Website: www.addaction.org.uk
Provides help for people with drug and alcohol problems.

Relate
Head Office, Premier House
Carolina Court
Lakeside
Doncaster DN4 5RA
Tel.: 0300 100 1234
Website: www.relate.org.uk
Deals with issues concerning relationships. There are other Relate offices around the country and full details are supplied on the website.

Victim Support
National Centre Office
Hallam House
59–60 Hallam Street
London W1W 6JL
Tel.: 0845 30 30 900 (support line)
Website: www.victimsupport.org/
Provides assistance to people who are the victims of crime.

Further reading

Many books about traumatic stress have been published: some for academics, some for clinicians, and others for members of the general public. Here are just a few to get you started.

Bremner, J. D., *Does Stress Damage the Brain?* Norton, London, 2005.

Calhoun, L. and Tedeschi, R. (eds), *Handbook of Posttraumatic Growth.* Lawrence Erlbaum, Mahwah, NJ, 2006.

Foa, E., Keane, T. and Friedman, M. (eds), *Effective Treatments for PTSD.* Guilford Press, New York, 2000.

Harvey, J. and Pauwels, B. (eds), *Post-Traumatic Stress Theory.* Brunner/Mazel, Philadelphia, PA, 2000.

Herman, J., *Trauma and Recovery.* Basic Books, New York, 1992 (14th edn, 1997).

Hunt, N., *Memory, War and Trauma.* Cambridge University Press, Cambridge, 2010.

Hunt, N. and McHale, S., *Understanding Traumatic Stress.* Sheldon, London, 2010.

Joseph, S., Williams, R. and Yule, W., *Understanding Post-traumatic Stress: A psychosocial perspective on PTSD and treatment.* Wiley-Blackwell, Oxford, 1992.

Resick, P., *Stress and Trauma.* Psychology Press, London, 2001.

Scott, M., *Moving on After Trauma.* Routledge, Abingdon, 2007.

Yule, W. (ed.), *Post-Traumatic Stress Disorders.* Wiley, Hoboken, NY, 1999.

Index